QUALITY MEDICAL EDITING

FOR THE HEALTHCARE DOCUMENTATION SPECIALIST

QUALITY MEDICAL EDITING

FOR THE HEALTHCARE DOCUMENTATION SPECIALIST

PATRICIA A. IRELAND, CMT, AHDI-F
MULTISPECIALTY CERTIFIED MEDICAL TRANSCRIPTIONIST,
INSTRUCTOR, MEDICAL/TECHNICAL AUTHOR AND EDITOR
SAN ANTONIO, TEXAS

KRISTIN M. WALL, CHDS, AHDI-F
CERTIFIED HEALTHCARE DOCUMENTATION SPECIALIST, AUTHOR,
PROFESSIONAL AND FREELANCE TECHNICAL EDITOR
FLEMING ISLAND, FLORIDA

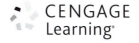

CENGAGE
Learning®

Australia • Brazil • Mexico • Singapore • United Kingdom • United States

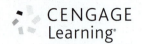

Quality Medical Editing for the Healthcare Documentation Specialist, First Edition
Patricia A. Ireland, Kristin M. Wall

SVP, GM Skills & Global Product Management:
Dawn Gerrain

Product Director: Matthew Seeley

Product Manager: Jadin Kavanaugh

Senior Director, Development:
Marah Bellegarde

Senior Production Director: Wendy Troeger

Production Director: Andrew Crouth

Product Development Manager: Juliet Steiner

Content Developer: Lauren Whalen

Product Assistant: Mark Turner

Vice President, Marketing Services:
Jennifer Ann Baker

Marketing Manager: Jonathan Sheehan

CL Mfg Planner: Breslin Beverly

Art and Cover Direction, Production
Management, and Composition:
Lumina Datamatics, Ltd.

Cover image(s): © LuminaStock/Thinkstockcom;
© cristovao/Shutterstock.com; © Monkey
Business Images/Shutterstock.com

Library of Congress Control Number: 2015930913

Book Only ISBN: 978-1-285-18706-8

Package ISBN: 978-1-285-18652-8

Cengage Learning
20 Channel Center Street
Boston, MA 02210
USA

Cengage Learning is a leading provider of customized learning solutions with employees residing in nearly 40 different countries and sales in more than 125 countries around the world. Find your local representative at **www.cengage.com**

Cengage Learning products are represented in Canada by Nelson Education, Ltd.

To learn more about Cengage Learning, visit **www.cengage.com**

Purchase any of our products at your local college store or at our preferred online store **www.cengagebrain.com**

Notice to the Reader

Publisher does not warrant or guarantee any of the products described herein or perform any independent analysis in connection with any of the product information contained herein. Publisher does not assume, and expressly disclaims, any obligation to obtain and include information other than that provided to it by the manufacturer. The reader is expressly warned to consider and adopt all safety precautions that might be indicated by the activities described herein and to avoid all potential hazards. By following the instructions contained herein, the reader willingly assumes all risks in connection with such instructions. The publisher makes no representations or warranties of any kind, including but not limited to, the warranties of fitness for particular purpose or merchantability, nor are any such representations implied with respect to the material set forth herein, and the publisher takes no responsibility with respect to such material. The publisher shall not be liable for any special, consequential, or exemplary damages resulting, in whole or part, from the readers' use of, or reliance upon, this material.

Printed in the United States of America
Print Number: 01   Print Year: 2015

"Nothing has really happened until it has been recorded."

Virginia Woolf, English author and critic (1882–1941)

DEDICATION

"One child, one teacher, one book, and one pen can change the world." – Malala Yousafzai

Malala Yousafzai, a 16-year-old student who survived being shot by the Taliban in 2012 after speaking out in favor of girls' education in Pakistan.

TABLE OF CONTENTS

FOREWORD

Back when transcription was done on typewriters and computers were so large they took up more space than the average Apple store of today, someone told me not to go into medical transcription. "They've got these computers that can type everything the doctor says," I was told. "You'll be obsolete in less than two years!"

Now, more than 30 years later, we carry the Internet in our pockets on smartphones, and speech recognition technology is everywhere. Technology sales hype promises of quick, effortless computer transcription of your dictated thoughts. But anyone who has used speech recognition on a smartphone knows how inaccurate those speech-recognized documents can be and how easy it is to miss some of those mistakes when you try to proofread them.

You want proof that a professional healthcare documentation specialist (HDS) should be looking at your speech-recognized medical records? Google "the dropped no." In this case presented by the Agency for Healthcare Research and Quality (AHRQ), a radiologist's ultrasound report erroneously indicated a deep venous thrombosis where none existed. The error was caused by the recording's failure to pick up the first word dictated, which was "no." The patient had unnecessary surgery to prevent damage from the nonexistent DVT.

Today, more and more HDSs find themselves not transcribing but rather editing speech-recognized text. Though this saves their fingers the stress of beating on keyboards, they need to develop a different mindset from that of straight transcribing to be successful. Instead of processing audio with one's hands, the SR editor reviews words while listening to audio. The difference is that words presented by the system can be seductive—the mind wants to hear what the eyes read. This means that the SR editor needs strong critical thinking abilities and deep medical knowledge to know when something's not right.

That is what authors Patricia Ireland and Kristin Wall strive to present in *Quality Medical Editing for the Healthcare Documentation Specialist*. Ireland, coauthor of the *Hillcrest Medical Center, Forrest General Medical Center* and *The Dictated Word* texts, and Wall, AHDI's senior programs coordinator, editor-in-chief of *Plexus* magazine, and coauthor of the *CMT Exam Guide*, are well qualified to teach the art of speech recognition editing. Though many transcription textbooks exist, this is the first text ever to focus on the skill of speech recognition editing.

As healthcare documentation specialists move increasingly into the world of SR editing, their roles in patient safety continue to be vital. The challenge for HDSs is to ensure that the words the clinician intends are the ones that end up in the patient's medical record.

Whether you are an experienced transcriptionist looking to increase your skills or a brand-new student starting from scratch in healthcare documentation, you'll find information that you will need in this book. *Quality Medical Editing* is an excellent introduction into the art of editing clinicians' SR drafts, which is a skill that future HDSs must embrace as the guardians of health record integrity.

Susan D. Dooley, MHA, CMT, AHDI-F

Susan D. Dooley, MHA, CMT, AHDI-F, has taught college-level medical transcription and healthcare core courses for more than 23 years. A professor at Seminole State College of Florida, she is the 2014–2015 president of the National Leadership Board of the Association for Healthcare Documentation Integrity (AHDI).

PREFACE

INTRODUCTION

Quality Medical Editing for the Healthcare Documentation Specialist has been written to provide training in medical editing for the healthcare documentation specialist (HDS) in community colleges, four-year colleges and universities, proprietary institutions, hospital in-service education, and medical transcription service organization (MTSO) training programs. This text would be useful in cross-training or retraining the newly employed HDS in medical editing. It would also serve military veterans and their spouses, the disabled and their caregivers, as well as retirees who have a background in healthcare and are looking for a new career.

WHY WE WROTE THIS TEXT

Quality Medical Editing was conceived because no medical editing texts existed. In searching the field, this was a void. In asking MTSOs, they were looking for help in training their employees. In asking instructors, they were looking for medical editing material to use in the classroom and in online programs. The time for *Quality Medical Editing* is now: QME for you and ME!

ORGANIZATION OF THE TEXT

Quality Medical Editing is organized into three units. Unit 1 discusses career and professional development including credentialing. Medical editing as a career is also covered and includes opportunities for career advancement and recommendations of continuing education. Unit 2 highlights important listening skills that are vital to the career of the medical editor. This includes tips for deciphering different accents and how to identify tricky medication usages, spellings, and sound-alikes. The unit concludes with a chapter that describes the differences between front-end and back-end speech recognition software. Unit 3 expands on the elements of medical editing and the skills needed to be a successful medical editor. This unit helps build professional skills such as keyboarding, ensuring accuracy, proofreading, and quality assurance.

Unit 4 goes even deeper into the specifics of the medical editing and provides examples of a variety of report types the health documentation specialist will encounter: correspondence, radiology, acute care, and chronic care. In addition to providing model reports for the medical editor to review and become familiar with, Unit 4 also includes 266 test reports representative of the types of VRS-generated reports a medical editor might encounter on the job. Students are asked to review these reports and identify any errors to be corrected.

Quality Medical Editing also includes a variety of appendices intended to enhance the student's learning experience. These appendices include an index of QME dictating healthcare professionals; challenging words, terms, and prefixes; list of drugs that includes trade names with corresponding generic names and treatment uses, *Do Not Use* list from The Joint Commission; postal service addressing standards; and a list of United States military bases.

Features

Quality Medical Editing includes a wide variety of features intended to prepare healthcare documentation specialists for a career in medical editing:

- Professional development discussion to include medical editing as a career
- Difficulties encountered in listening to accented dictation, medications, and sound-alikes
- Front-end versus back-end speech recognition definitions and explanations

- Elements of medical editing to include the mechanics, accuracy, and quality assurance
- Critical thinking scenarios in Chapters 7, 8, 9, and 10
- Challenging words, terms, and prefixes in Appendix B
- Robust list of trade names with corresponding generic names of drugs in Appendix C
- Web links to real-life medical procedures in Appendix G

ANCILLARY PACKAGE

The complete supplement package for *Quality Medical Editing for the Healthcare Documentation Specialist* was developed to achieve two goals:

1. To assist students in learning and applying the information presented in the text.
2. To assist instructors in planning and implementing their courses in the most efficient manner as well as to provide exceptional resources to enhance their students' experience.

Student Premium Website

This password-protected website is designed to maximize learning while providing a multimedia approach to understanding the concepts presented in this text. Follow the directions on the printed access card to log on at http://www.cengagebrain.com. In the student resources you will find:

- A total of 266 medical reports associated with the activities listed in Unit 4. These reports cover correspondence, radiology, acute care, and chronic care. The reports are intended for students to review and correct errors.
- Dictation audio files associated with each of the 266 medical report activities. Students can refer to these audio files as they review the medical reports.

Instructor Companion Website

ISBN 13: 978-1-285-18790-7

Spend less time planning and more time teaching with Cengage Learning's Instructor Resources to accompany *Quality Medical Editing for the Healthcare Documentation Specialist*. The Instructor Companion Website can be accessed by going to http://www.cengage.com/login to create a unique user log-in. The password-protected Instructor Resources include the following:

- Test Bank with quizzes for use as homework, classroom work, and testing material
- Test Report Solutions for Unit 4 activities
- "Snippet" dictation activities and answer keys
- Answer keys for all quizzes and critical thinking activities in the core text and instructor resources
- PowerPoint presentation on grammar/punctuation and research techniques with quizzes

ABOUT THE AUTHORS

Patricia A. Ireland, CMT, AHDI-F, has been active in the field of medical transcription since 1968, both as a multispecialty practitioner and as an instructor. She lives in San Antonio, Texas, working as a freelance medical/technical author and editor. She has been a medical transcription instructor since the 1970s, teaching online medical transcription programs since 2000. She has co-authored three medical transcription textbooks, this being her fourth. Ms. Ireland encourages questions and comments about this text and can be reached at pat.ireland68@yahoo.com.

Kristin M. Wall, CHDS, AHDI-F, has over 16 years' experience in the healthcare documentation industry as an acute care practitioner and in her current role as senior programs coordinator at the Association for Healthcare Documentation Integrity (AHDI) and editor-in-chief of *Plexus* magazine. She co-authored the *CMT Exam Guide: A Walk Through the Blue Print*. Having a meticulous eye for detail, she is a freelance copyeditor for numerous medical transcription and style-related texts as well as fiction books. She enjoys mentoring and "paying it forward" and has been a speaker at a variety of local, state, and national AHDI conferences and credentialing study groups. Ms. Wall can be reached at Kris@EFIalchemy.com.

ACKNOWLEDGEMENTS

We deeply appreciate the assistance of all those at Cengage Learning who helped in the production of *Quality Medical Editing*.

Our particular thanks go to the following professionals for their advice, review, and mentorship:

Jerrie Bolton, Healthcare Documentation Specialist, Galveston, TX

Carol Crumrine, Medical Transcriptionist, Columbia, NJ

Susan Dooley, MHA, CMT, AHDI-F, Sorrento, FL

Linda Galbraith, Healthcare Documentation Specialist, Foley, AL

Judy Matos, Healthcare Documentation Specialist, Sandy Hook, CT

Stacey L. McFarlin, Consolidated Computing Solutions, San Antonio, TX

Sherry L. Martin, CMT, AHDI-F, Transcription Manager, Jacksonville, FL

Rebecca McSwain, PhD, CHDS, Tucson, AZ

Julie Naimi, Healthcare Documentation Specialist, Ft. Lauderdale, FL

Marge Parker, Healthcare Documentation Specialist, Hayes, VA

Lea M. Sims, CHDS, AHDI-F, Jacksonville, FL

Diane Smith, CMT, Gatesville, TX

Carmen Tyler, BS, Parma, OH

Reviewers

Cindi Brassington, MS, CMA

Susan D. Dooley, MHA, CMT, AHDI-F

Deborah Huber

Cheryl A Miller, MBA/HCM

Robin Minter, CHDS, AHDI-F, CMSS

Charlene Thiessen, CMT, AHDI-F, MEd

QUALITY MEDICAL EDITING

FOR THE HEALTHCARE DOCUMENTATION SPECIALIST

UNIT 1

CAREER DEVELOPMENT

CHAPTER 1

PROFESSIONAL DEVELOPMENT

KEY TERMS

abstractor
American Association for Medical Transcription (AAMT)
American Health Information Management Association (AHIMA)
American Medical Association (AMA)
Association for Healthcare Documentation Integrity (AHDI)
automated speech recognition (ASR)
Certified Healthcare Documentation Specialist (CHDS)
Certified Medical Transcriptionist (CMT)
Clinical Documentation Industry Association (CDIA)
continuing education credits (CECs)
continuous speech recognition (CSR)
Credential Qualifying Examination (CQE)
database
electronic voice recognition translation (EVRT)
end user
healthcare documentation specialist (HDS)
Health Information and Management Systems Society (HIMSS)

Health Level Seven (HL7)
Health Story Project (HSP)
high reliability
job classification
medical editing
medical editor (ME)
medical transcriptionist (MT)
networking
proctored examination
professional association
quality assurance (QA)
Registered Healthcare Documentation Specialist (RHDS)
Registered Medical Transcriptionist (RMT)
regulatory agencies
sentinel event
speech recognition engine (SRE)
speech recognition technology (SRT)
straight transcription
The Joint Commission (TJC)
traditional transcription
verbatim
voice recognition engine (VRE)

LEARNING OBJECTIVES

1. Understand the difference between traditional transcription and speech recognition editing.

2. Explain the difference between front-end versus back-end speech recognition.

3. Learn ways in which building knowledge is beneficial to job performance outcomes.

4. Define what a professional association is and the role it plays.

5. Learn about the Association for Healthcare Documentation Integrity and how professional associations can work together.

6. Understand what credentials are and why they are important.

7. Discover what credentials are available in healthcare documentation and how to become credentialed.

INTRODUCTION

Traditional transcription—also called **straight transcription**—is the term used to describe work performed in which blank pages are filled with words transcribed based on voice file recordings of patient medical encounters dictated by clinicians. Transcription is based on the interpretation of what the originator of the medical report or correspondence is saying using knowledge, experience, and reliable resources to ensure accuracy of the report. This transcribed text is then proofread, edited as needed, and in some cases sent to the **quality assurance (QA)** department for feedback, verification of information, or correction. Finally, the completed document is forwarded not only to a **database** but also to the **end user**, such as a hospital unit or physician practice.

Healthcare documentation specialist (HDS) is an umbrella term that encompasses various titles of different types of jobs performed within the realm of medical record documentation. Examples of other titles include **medical transcriptionist (MT)**, **medical editor (ME)**, **abstractor**, voice recognition editor, and speech recognition editor.

N.B.: For the purposes of this text, "healthcare documentation specialist" or "HDS" will be used as the universal term.

Medical editing is the term used to describe work performed by an HDS after receiving the medical report already filled with words inserted by a **speech recognition engine (SRE)**—also called **automated speech recognition (ASR)**, and **continuous speech recognition (CSR), electronic voice recognition translation (EVRT)**, and **voice recognition engine (VRE)**—based on how the electronic equipment interprets the speech of the originator of the medical report. The HDS must edit the document while listening to the originator's corresponding voice file. Some may conclude that the latter scenario is easier—after all, the original words are already there, right? On the contrary, the challenge for a speech recognition editor is the ability to successfully interpret what the ears hear against what the eyes see and the brain knows in order to identify errors in a speech-recognized document. Although the physical demands are typically decreased in performing speech-recognized editing versus traditional transcription, in which there is much more keyboarding of a report start to finish, the mental demands on the HDS to focus and concentrate are increased in SR editing.

N.B.: For the purposes of this text, "speech recognition" or "SR" will be used as the universal term.

Quality Medical Editing is designed to not only train the new HDS in SR editing but also to help the experienced HDS master this new skill set.

KNOWLEDGE IS POWER

To paraphrase Jordan Phoenix, author of the blog "Uncommon Sense for 21st Century Living," most people have heard the phrase "knowledge is power." However, many may not truly understand it or know how to use it to improve lives. Phoenix states: "Knowledge = Options = Power."

To educate ourselves is to learn new things—new knowledge, previously unknown. The more educated we are, the better our ability to make well-informed decisions for ourselves and those around us. In turn, we become more valuable people. Phoenix goes on to state: "The more valuable of a person you are, the more people will want to be around you, the more they will want to work with you, the more they introduce you to others who need your help or can help you, and the more doors and opportunities open in your life."

Knowledge is something that no one can take away from us. We are in charge of our own destiny and our own path to reach that destiny.

Another catch-phrase sometimes heard is "you don't know what you don't know." Although this may seem like a "catch-22," just think it over. In new situations, we are aware of what we do not know. But throughout life, we can remain blissfully unaware of vast areas of knowledge that simply have never been brought to our attention—about which we never even wondered.

A person's knowledge (what is in his or her brain) is key. It's true that HDSs must know how to research well and be able to decipher reliable online resources from the copious amounts of misinformation floating around the web. It's also true that tools such as spellcheckers and word expander programs make HDSs' lives *much* easier, but we each must become our own resource. Here's why: The more we know . . .

- the more efficient we will be.
- the faster we will be able to complete our work.
- the less time we will spend researching.

- the more valuable we become as employees or contractors.
- the better resources we are to others.
- the bigger our incomes can become.
- the better we will be at passing credentialing exams or employment tests—either to get hired or to get a promotion.

Electronic tools should be used to contribute to the efficiency and accuracy in documentation, but human intelligence cannot be replaced by machines and software. Therefore, do not become complacent or lazy, relying too heavily on electronic crutches (text expanders and spellcheck). Do not "tune out" or go on "autopilot" while transcribing or editing patient reports. This is when mistakes can happen. Even pilots and ship captains have been criticized for relying too heavily on actual autopilot; this has been blamed for some major airline and boating accidents.

It is necessary to stay alert, focused, and tuned *in* to what is heard and seen on the computer screen. Always question whether the information makes sense in context and evaluate how inconsistencies should be handled. Does your employer or client follow strict **verbatim** guidelines, or are HDSs allowed to use their critical thinking skills and common sense to edit verifiable information? Know the protocol outlined by each employer or client for how to deal with such matters. Knowledge is power—use it to make HDSs and their work more indispensable.

PROFESSIONAL ORGANIZATIONS

What Is a Professional Organization?

A **professional association** is most often a not-for-profit organization that acts to protect the public by maintaining and upholding standards of training and ethics in their profession. Associations typically develop and monitor educational programs; provide continuing education modalities; and often, but not always, offer certification. Associations may put out position statements and advocate on behalf of their industry.

What Is the Role of a Professional Association within an Industry?

A professional association exists to elevate, educate, and empower the professionals within it to make sound choices on their own. It exists to be watchful of trends and changes within the industry and to impart that information to its members. It exists to promote excellence in education, practice, and compensation within the profession. It can make strong recommendations and urge leadership within the industry to embrace high standards, but it cannot force individuals to do so. The role of an association is to empower its professionals, not to control the industry or restrict the free trade of services within it.

About the Association for Healthcare Documentation Integrity

As noted at the website (www.ahdionline.org), the **Association for Healthcare Documentation Integrity (AHDI)**, formerly the **American Association for Medical Transcription (AAMT)**, "is the world's largest professional society representing the clinical documentation sector." AHDI is a not-for-profit 501(c) professional association. Unlike unions who have legal authority to intervene in labor disputes between professionals and their employees, AHDI is not a policing or regulatory organization, nor would it be legally allowed to operate as such. AHDI's purpose is to "set and uphold standards for education and practice in the field of health data capture and documentation that ensure the highest level of accuracy, privacy, and security for the U.S. healthcare system in order to protect public health, increase patient safety, and improve quality of care for healthcare consumers. AHDI works to advocate for workforce development and credentialing in allied health and the critical role of technology-enabled documentation knowledge worker in the electronic health record (EHR)."

AAMT was established in 1978 as part of an effort to achieve recognition for the medical transcription profession. In the beginning, the association focused on educating medical professionals about what medical transcriptionists do and how their work affects the quality of health care. When the U.S. Department of Labor granted medical transcriptionists their own **job classification** in 1999, it was an important milestone to getting the work recognized as much more than clerical. In 2012, AHDI adopted a new title—healthcare documentation specialists—to reflect the broad and extensive responsibilities and services they provide in the creation of accurate and comprehensive patient care records.

Today, AHDI continues to champion excellence in healthcare documentation and advance patient safety through the precise capture of the patient's health story. AHDI helps protect patient health information through continuous workforce development and the support of practitioners and industry partners.

AHDI works tirelessly to give thousands of healthcare documentation specialists a voice before legislative and **regulatory agencies** and to ensure they are recognized for their contributions to patient safety and risk management.

What Are the Benefits of Belonging to a Professional Organization?

Joining a professional association within your field can enhance your career, knowledge, and skills. **Networking** is one excellent benefit. Developing relationships with like-minded professionals about relatable topics provides people to turn to when questions or concerns arise. It allows for opportunities of professional growth and of sharing knowledge with others. Think of networking like a popular story or video posted on Facebook going viral. A person may share that story or video with a hundred Facebook friends, maybe 25 of those friends repost the story or video on their Facebook page, being seen by their 250 friends, some of whom will share it also, and so the cycle continues. Sometimes you even see a story or video on Facebook but *don't* share it, yet days, weeks, or months later you may see the same story or video shared by a different friend in a different state who has no connection to the person of the original post. This highlights how fast and widespread people are making connections—in one way or another—each and every day. Many times, the relationships you foster through professional associations lead to lifelong friendships.

Career resources are another great offering by most associations—things such as:

1. Job board or forum showing the latest openings.
2. Print or online publications, such as member magazines and newsletters.
3. Matching of mentors with mentees.
4. Discounts on goods and services, including for students.

Resources such as these provide education via multiple vehicles, which allow you to learn at your own pace and stay informed of the latest trends and happenings within the association and the industry. In our fast-paced, time-constricted lives, this is an efficient way to receive valuable information without much effort.

Associations Working Together

Within a given career field, multiple associations may represent the many types of professionals working in that field. Take health care, for example: Numerous nursing associations exist for the various types of nurses (critical care nurses, student nurses, emergency nurses, holistic nurses, nurse practitioners, and so on). Multiple associations exist for physicians—the most common being the **American Medical Association (AMA)**, although, again, there is an abundance of associations for the myriad medical specialties—which is a good thing, by the way! The more focused an association can be on a specific area of an industry, the more its members will benefit by having catered information, news, and resources for what those practitioners need as opposed to having to wade through materials and information of little or no relevance.

Often it is to the benefit of two or more associations to collaborate on joint projects or initiatives that would benefit the workforce or effect change regarding public outcomes of both or all involved. This can save time and money and can bring together groups of people of varying backgrounds, experiences, and ideas to work on a common goal.

AHDI has collaborated with varying organizations, such as the **American Health Information Management Association (AHIMA)**, **Health Story Project (HSP)**, **Health Level Seven (HL7)**, **Health Information and Management Systems Society (HIMSS)**, and the former **Clinical Documentation Industry Association (CDIA)**, among others. These associations have worked together for the common good, creating best practices, industry standards and guidelines, and optimizing healthcare outcomes using information technology.

The Joint Commission (TJC) is an independent, not-for-profit organization that accredits and certifies more than 20,500 healthcare organizations and programs in the United States. TJC also develops standards related to patient safety and quality of care. TJC's mission is "to continuously improve health care for the public, in collaboration with other stakeholders, by evaluating healthcare organizations and inspiring them to excel in providing safe and effective care of the highest quality and value." TJC has outlined a number of National Patient Safety Goals (found on its website, http://www.jointcommission.org). These goals include numerous patient safety and performance measurement fact sheets outlining how to identify and address emerging patient safety issues in a wide variety of healthcare settings. The fact sheets provide protocols and processes for topics such as patient-centered communications, the official "Do Not Use" list of abbreviations, quality checks and quality reports, accountability measures, and much more.

A big part of what TJC does is to investigate sentinel events. A **sentinel event** is "an unexpected death or serious physical—including loss of limb or function—or psychological injury, or the risk thereof." TJC works with the healthcare organizations, which are expected to complete a root cause analysis (typically caused by human factors, communication breakdown, or leadership failure) of the organization's systems and processes in order to make improvements, to reduce risk, and to monitor the effectiveness of those improvements. An interesting side note is that according to The Joint Commission, the reporting of most sentinel events to TJC by healthcare organizations is voluntary and represents only a small portion of actual events that occur.

TJC also teaches principles of **high reliability**—ways of maintaining consistently high levels of safety and quality over time and across all healthcare services and settings. This model outlines three requirements for achieving high reliability:

1. Leadership—Leaders must make a commitment to the goal of high reliability.
2. Safety culture—The organizational culture that supports high reliability must be fully implemented.
3. Robust Process Improvement—The tools of robust process improvement must be adopted.

Each health professional's role contributes to high reliability. Evidence suggests that the risk of errors in health care harmful to patients may be increasing. New devices, procedures, medications, and equipment are constantly being added to the mix. These complexities greatly increase the likelihood of errors. The HDS is part of the risk management team in health care, helping to identify and correct errors in the record. These steps improve patient care and safety; as such, the attention to detail brought by the HDS is what many dictating physicians rely on.

CREDENTIALING

What Are Credentials?

As noted in *Merriam-Webster*, a credential is "(1) a quality, skill, or experience that makes a person suited to do a job, and (2) a document which shows that a person is qualified to do a particular job." In healthcare documentation and editing, one's temperament and discipline, along with skills and experience acquired through formal education, exposure, and on-the-job training, as well as ongoing continuing education are the combined foundational elements that say to employers, clients, and peers, "I am competent and qualified to perform this work." Becoming registered or certified is the process by which a person is tested on their knowledge and skills as well as the standards and best practices for their chosen field.

In healthcare documentation and editing, AHDI is the only professional organization that offers credentialing and by which a healthcare documentation specialist can become registered or certified. Some colleges and trade schools offer healthcare documentation and editing programs after which a certificate of completion is issued. This indicates only successful completion of said program, not that the student has been registered or certified by examination through AHDI.

Why Is Credentialing Important?

Credentialing is a measurable way to help ensure that only skilled, qualified, and accountable individuals have access to patient records for the purpose of creating, modifying, and formatting the clinical care record—a legal document.

Promoting a credentialing requirement for the profession will send a clear message to healthcare providers that HDSs have met minimum standards to engage in a risk management role.

What Are the Benefits of Being Credentialed?

The following are common attributes of credentialed professionals found throughout any industry, including those in the healthcare spectrum. Although becoming credentialed is voluntary, it shows job readiness and level-specific competency to prospective employers, clients, and industry colleagues.

Credentialed professionals are:

- Seen as just that—a professional and a valued member of the healthcare team.
- Shown respect; one way this can be demonstrated is by having his or her opinion valued and sought out.
- Trained in Health Insurance Portability and Accountability Act (HIPAA) compliance, privacy, and security, among other best practices and standards in the industry.

- Continual learners who enjoy building their knowledge and skills.
- Self-confident in their careers, taking pride in their work.
- Often promoted and given more responsibility than noncredentialed personnel.
- Often paid more, provided additional benefits, and reimbursed the cost of examination and **continuing education credits (CECs)** by their employers.
- Marketable in the healthcare documentation industry.
- Readily identified and recognized by their peers and the public because of the initials placed after their names.

What Credentials Are Offered in Healthcare Documentation?

In 2013, AHDI rebranded the credentialing exams to both better align with their name and to reflect the expanded skill-set competencies noted on the additional blueprint domains. Thus, there are four recognized credentials in healthcare documentation, also called medical transcription. These include:

- Registered Medical Transcriptionist (RMT)
- Certified Medical Transcriptionist (CMT)
- Registered Healthcare Documentation Specialist (RHDS)
- Certified Healthcare Documentation Specialist (CHDS)

A **Registered Medical Transcriptionist (RMT)** is a healthcare documentation specialist who earned his or her credential as a recent graduate of a medical transcription program, with fewer than two years' experience in acute care, or who works in a single-specialty environment. An RMT's scope of knowledge as assessed through core competencies on examination including English and grammar, medical terminology, pharmacology, anatomy and physiology, disease processes, basic laboratory and radiologic terminology and normal values, and knowledge and application of styles and standards according to *The Book of Style for Medical Transcription,* 3rd edition.

RMTs recredential every three years by successfully completing a recredentialing course through AHDI. The RMT credential is still valid; but an examination for the RMT credential is no longer offered by AHDI, and all who hold the RMT credential will earn the RHDS credential upon successful completion of the RHDS Recredentialing Course at the end of their cycles. RMTs do have the option to take the RHDS Recredentialing Course at any time in their cycles to earn the RHDS credential earlier. The RMT credential will naturally sunset over time.

A **Registered Healthcare Documentation Specialist (RHDS)** is a healthcare documentation specialist who earned his or her credential as a recent graduate of a medical transcription program, with fewer than two years' experience in acute care, or who works in a single-specialty environment. An RHDS's scope of knowledge as assessed through core competencies on examination include all items previously named on the RMT examination (English and grammar, medical terminology, pharmacology, anatomy and physiology, disease processes, basic laboratory and radiologic terminology and normal values, and knowledge and application of styles and standards according to *The Book of Style for Medical Transcription,* 3rd edition) plus basic editing and flagging of reports, identifying protected health information (PHI) and HIPAA privacy and security rules, common Joint Commission and Department of Health and Human Services (DHHS) rules and regulations, common computer technology terminology, abbreviations, and meanings, as well as common health information technology data exchange terminology, abbreviations, and meanings.

The RHDS exam tests the knowledge and skills of candidates through multiple-choice questions and transcription of one or more blanks representing omitted information while listening to audio clips.

RHDSs recredential every three years by successfully completing a recredentialing course through AHDI. At any time, an RHDS may opt to sit for the CHDS exam if he or she feels well prepared and meets criteria outlined. If the candidate passes, his or her RHDS credential would be relinquished in favor of the CHDS credential, and a new recertification cycle for the person's CHDS would begin. If the candidate does not pass, the current cycle as an RHDS would continue and he or she would need to meet the recredentialing requirements in order to maintain his or her RHDS status. Of note, having first earned the RHDS credential is a prerequisite to being eligible to take the CHDS exam.

A **Certified Medical Transcriptionist (CMT)** is a healthcare documentation specialist with a minimum of two years' experience in acute care or multispecialty equivalent who earned his or her credential through successful completion of the CMT examination. A CMT's scope of knowledge as assessed through core competencies on examination includes expansive English and grammar, proficiency in most report types and medical specialties, comprehensive medical terminology, comprehensive pharmacology, comprehensive anatomy and physiology, thorough knowledge of disease processes, intensive editing and QA, in-depth surgical and operative terminology knowledge and comprehension, and in-depth knowledge and application of styles and standards according to *The Book of Style for Medical Transcription,* 3rd edition.

CMTs recredential every three years by earning a minimum of 30 CECs during that time period. At least 24 CECs must be earned in the four core areas of *Clinical Medicine, Medical Transcription Tools, Technology and the Workplace,* and *Medicolegal Issues.* The remaining 6 required CECs may be obtained in either the core areas mentioned above or the two optional areas of *Complementary Medicine* and *Professional Development.*

CMTs are not required to pursue the CHDS credential (doing so is optional and voluntary). AHDI continues to service the CMT credential under its current recredentialing program requirements, although an examination for the CMT credential is no longer offered by AHDI. CMTs have the option to take the CHDS Bridge Course to earn the CHDS credential.

A **Certified Healthcare Documentation Specialist (CHDS)** is a healthcare documentation specialist with a minimum of two years' experience in acute care or multispecialty equivalent who earns his or her credential through successful completion of the CHDS examination. A CHDS's scope of knowledge as assessed through core competencies on examination includes all areas previously noted (expansive English and grammar, proficient in most report types and medical specialties, comprehensive medical terminology, comprehensive pharmacology, comprehensive anatomy and physiology, thorough knowledge of disease processes, intensive editing and QA, in-depth surgical and operative terminology knowledge and comprehension, and in-depth knowledge and application of styles and standards (according to *The Book of Style for Medical Transcription,* 3rd edition) plus extensive knowledge of PHI and HIPAA privacy and security rules and regulations; extensive knowledge of TJC and DHHS rules and regulations; extensive knowledge of computer technology terminology, abbreviations, and definitions; extensive knowledge of health information

technology and data exchange terminology, abbreviations, and definitions; extensive knowledge and comprehension of EHRs and electronic medical records (EMRs), EMR terminology and definitions; and extensive knowledge and comprehension of speech recognition technology and natural language processing terminology and definitions.

The CHDS exam tests the knowledge and skills of candidates through multiple-choice questions, transcription of one or more blanks representing omitted information while listening to audio clips, and **speech recognition technology (SRT)** editing in which candidates are provided with a speech-recognized draft of text and the dictated audio clips. Candidates must identify the word or phrase captured in error by the SRT engine and transcribe the correct word or phrase.

CHDSs recredential every three years by earning a minimum of 30 CECs during that time period. At least 24 CECs must be earned in the four core areas of *Clinical Medicine, Medical Transcription Tools, Technology and the Workplace,* and *Medicolegal Issues.* The remaining 6 required CECs may be obtained in either the core areas mentioned above or the two optional areas of *Complementary Medicine* and *Professional Development.*

How Does One Become Credentialed?

Registered Healthcare Documentation Specialist Examination

Entry-level healthcare documentation specialists (with fewer than two years' acute care experience) or those working in a single-specialty environment who desire to sit for the RHDS examination should visit the AHDI website to review all criteria and information related to the RHDS.

Candidates should also read the *Credentialing Candidate Guide* in full. This guide contains in-depth information about the credentialing process, test development and delivery, eligibility requirements, content focus, RHDS exam blue print, technology requirements, sample RHDS content questions, transcription against audio details, and frequently asked questions (FAQs).

Certified Healthcare Documentation Specialist Examination

Seasoned HDSs with at least two years' acute care (or multispecialty equivalent) experience who desire to sit for the CHDS examination should visit the AHDI website to review all criteria and information related to the CHDS. Of note, candidates must already possess the RHDS credential to be eligible to sit for the CHDS exam.

Candidates should also read the *Credentialing Candidate Guide* in full. This guide contains in-depth information about the credentialing process, test development and delivery, eligibility requirements, content focus, CHDS exam blue print, technology requirements, sample CHDS content questions, transcription against audio details, and FAQs.

Credential Qualifying Examination

Seasoned HDSs with at least two years' acute care (or multispecialty equivalent) experience who desire to sit for the CHDS examination but who *do not* already possess the RHDS credential may choose to take the **Credential Qualifying Examination (CQE)**, which allows the candidate to test on both RHDS and CHDS content in a single exam session. Candidates who successfully pass the RHDS exam portion will have earned the RHDS credential and will go on to take the CHDS exam portion. If the CHDS exam portion is also successfully completed, the candidate will have earned the CHDS credential (thus relinquishing the RHDS credential; both credentials would not be used). The CQE is available only at Onsite Testing Centers and is not available as an online **proctored examination**.

CHAPTER 2

MEDICAL EDITING AS A CAREER

KEY TERMS

apprenticeship
externship
hearing acuity
internship

medical transcription service organization (MTSOs)
return on investment (ROI)
vested interest

LEARNING OBJECTIVES

1. List the main differences between the healthcare documentation specialist (HDS) skill set and the medical editor skill set.

2. Identify four potential areas of employment for an experienced HDS.

3. Explain the process by which schools become "Association for Healthcare Documentation Integrity (AHDI) approved."

4. Explain why attending an "AHDI-approved" school would benefit a student.

5. Identify the most effective kind of password.

6. List three ways to gain experience as a medical editor.

7. Review the 10 tips for job searching and interviewing.

INTRODUCTION

Independent classifications for medical editors and healthcare documentation specialists (HDSs) are not yet defined, thus providing no supporting employment or wage data at this time. These statistics are still captured for the title of medical transcriptionist (MT), standard occupational classification number 31-9094. According to the U.S. Bureau of Labor Statistics, the annual wage for an MT ranges from $22,750 to $47,960, with the median wage right at $34,590 ($16.36 per hour). This average median pay is on par with medical records and health information technicians as well as secretaries and administrative assistants: higher than receptionists, medical assistants, and information clerks and slightly lower than court reporters.

The job outlook is expected to grow 8% through the year 2022. Healthcare documentation remains an in-demand career field that is critical to patient safety and the integrity of medical documentation. It is a career best suited for those with an eye for detail and who can remain focused for long periods of time. It can be a very rewarding career choice for those who have a passion for the spoken and written word, combined with a love of the field of healthcare and enjoyment of technology.

EDUCATION

Medical editing of dictated medical records is an extension of the act of transcribing the original medical documents in a blank screen. The HDS, acting as medical editor, listens to the dictation and edits what has been recorded via the speech recognition engine. Special programs and keyboard applications are used in this process to help the HDS follow the dictation through the text. Medical editors must use vigilant attention and focus while editing as the eyes, ears, and brain work together to help ensure accuracy of the record. This is a bit of a different skill set from that used in traditional medical transcription, in which the HDS is producing transcribed text based on what he or she hears versus the brain processing and matching what the eyes see on the screen with what the ears hear during medical editing. After the document has been corrected with regard to accurate terminology and spelling, grammar, and necessary clarifications of the record, it is sent to the originating provider for signature.

People—from vendors and healthcare professionals to HDSs themselves—have been saying for years that our profession is going away. However, hospitals and **medical transcription service organizations (MTSOs)** are looking for full-time acute care HDSs in every nook and cranny, dredging their entire past databases.

Schools that teach healthcare documentation often have requests for more than 100 acute care-trained HDSs a year. Production companies want to hire acute care HDSs as well. Résumés have been requested everywhere imaginable—through résumé sites, email blasts, forums, social media, and so on. The vast majority of responses are from people who have experience only in clinic work—the chronic care setting.

What students may not fully realize is that clinic work in healthcare documentation is not always a viable long-term plan. The work is relatively simple and is the first to go offshore or to 100% speech recognition. Acute care healthcare documentation, however, is an acceptable standard for long-term success, and it remains in high demand. Those who chose to do clinical work are now looking to polish their skill set in order to be viable long-term HDSs in the acute care arena.

Although the myth of jobs being scarce likely will continue, those with acute care training will continue to enjoy their security and in-demand status as more and more clinic care-oriented HDSs realize that they need additional training to remain viable in a fast-moving industry. No, healthcare documentation is definitely not going away; however, those who enjoy this career field must upgrade their skills via continuing education to stay current and employable.

Other potential areas of employment for acute care HDSs include legal transcription, scribes, quality assurance (QA) professionals, trainers and facilitators, instructors, patient advocates, authors, and editors.

Quality Medical Editing is designed to be included as a semester in either a beginning MT or healthcare documentation program or an advanced MT or HDS program. It enhances the medical terminology, anatomy and physiology, pharmacology, laboratory and diagnostic studies, and Health Insurance Portability and Accountability Act (HIPAA) privacy and security classes that are normally taught. A good, solid education on which to build is an important start in a new career. From there, the HDS will gain experience through training and practice, which will lead to finding employment.

Healthcare documentation and editing programs can be completed at a brick-and-mortar facility, such as a local community college, or through an online program. The type of program you choose may be based on several factors, including:

- Preference of online learning or self-paced study versus an in-person learning environment.
- Availability of a healthcare documentation and editing program in your area.
- Flexibility in your schedule to attend classes during set times versus completing course work around your work and family schedules.
- Cost of the program.
- Quality and quantity of the program components and education being provided.

It is recommended to review the Association for Healthcare Documentation Integrity (AHDI) Model Curriculum for Healthcare Documentation to become familiar with what aspects should be covered in this type of program. Although offerings may vary from school to school, the foundational elements included in the model curriculum should be met in order for students to feel confident that they are getting a sound, well-rounded education in healthcare documentation in order to be employable as an entry-level HDS upon program completion. Such programs will assure consistency and high-quality outcomes for healthcare documentation education.

Program Approval

AHDI, in fact, has an Education Approval Program by which schools may submit their program specifications to be reviewed and either approved or denied if the program does not meet the set criteria. Programs must comply with specific educational and institutional criteria as established by AHDI. There is no formal accreditation process for healthcare documentation programs; however, the AHDI program approval is regarded by industry employers as an emerging benchmark for job-ready workforce candidates.

In May 2012, AHDI introduced the title of healthcare documentation specialist, as noted in Chapter 1. *The Model Curriculum for Healthcare Documentation*, 5th Edition, "affirms AHDI's commitment to the highest standards in education and training in healthcare documentation. The changes in healthcare information and documentation continue to offer new opportunities for well-educated, well-trained individuals; and this latest edition has been repurposed as an educational program for a broadly conceived suite of still-emerging roles under the label of healthcare documentation."

AHDI includes a listing of all approved schools on its website (http://www.ahdionline.org) as a convenience for those looking for a healthcare documentation program. These schools have been vigorously vetted through AHDI's Education Approval Program's review process. Schools that have met all criteria and requirements are considered "approved" and therefore allowed to list themselves as AHDI-Approved Programs. The AHDI website lists course type (campus-based versus online learning), type of enrollment (open or seasonal), and any funding options that may be available.

Whether you choose an onsite or online program, be sure to do your homework and compare all the facts before making the decision that is right for you. (Also see Appendix G for further resources.)

Return on Investment

When choosing a career path and making the decision to further your education, you have a **vested interest** in your future. The concept of getting a **return on investment (ROI)** means that the investor will yield some benefits. Having a high ROI means the gains are considerably favorable compared with the initial investment. It does not matter if you are just starting out, if you have decided to change careers, or if after retirement you feel you have more to offer. In essence, the more time and effort you invest in yourself— through focused education, training, and good decision making—the more favorable outcome (foundational knowledge and skills) and outlook (job prospects) you will reap. One of the best perks to pursuing a career as an HDS is that it can be done anywhere by anyone who has been properly trained and has a computer and Internet access.

GAINING EXPERIENCE

Guess what? By having completed at least a basic healthcare documentation program, worked in the healthcare documentation field, or begun *Quality Medical Editing*, you have already started gaining experience! Experience can come in the form of knowledge learned or skills acquired that give you a leg up and help you stand out from the crowd. The more initiative you take to learn, practice, and apply your knowledge and skills, the more of a sought-after asset you will be.

There are various ways to gain experience as a medical editor. Look for companies that offer an **internship**, an **externship**, or an **apprenticeship**. These opportunities can be a great way to gain access to editing platforms and site specifics while also learning dictators' speaking habits and accents.

Although it may be ideal, and even necessary, to work full-time, part-time opportunities can be useful to acquire the knowledge and skills you need in editing. It is a foot in the door that can lead to better opportunities or full-time employment after a period of time. Use such time to show initiative, learn all that you can, and prove your worth to your employer. Those who stand out against the crowd show their confidence and ability to shine. Employers will take notice.

If employment proves elusive initially, use that time to review books and resources from school; take further online courses to enhance your knowledge and practice editing using dictated voice files, such as those provided with this text. Remember, the language of medicine is like learning a foreign language: the more you are exposed to and understand that language, the more fluent you will become.

Job Skills, Knowledge, and Responsibilities

A wide array of job skills is required in healthcare documentation and medical editing, some of which may be acquired on the job. You should have at least a basic-to-intermediate level of knowledge and skills in the following areas:

Skills

- Operating and maintaining a personal computer and keeping the software current
- Word processing (e.g., Microsoft Office Suite)
- Researching and referencing via the Internet, books, and other resources
- Using electronic programs and resources such as email, word expanders, and instant messaging
- Thinking critically
- Paying attention to detail
- Concentrating, shutting out peripheral sounds while focusing on the job at hand
- **Hearing acuity** (refer to Unit 2, Chapter 3)

Knowledge

- Proper grammar and punctuation as it pertains to healthcare documentation
- HIPAA privacy and security rules and regulations
- Medical terminology
- Anatomy and physiology
- Pharmacology
- Laboratory medicine and diagnostic studies
- Healthcare records
- Technologies

Responsibilities

- Accurately editing medical records
- Verifying correct patient identifiers and dictator information
- Flagging reports
- Using the quality assurance (QA) system
- Understanding and applying HIPAA privacy and security rules and regulations
- As an employee, following your facility rules and regulations
- As an independent contractor (IC), treating all employees fairly
- As an IC, staying within city, county, and state laws
- As an IC, keeping files backed up appropriately and maintaining servers
- Choosing passwords of appropriate difficulty; keeping passwords updated regularly

N.B.: The above lists of skills, knowledge, and responsibilities are not all inclusive. All workers have a responsibility to perform their duties to the best of their abilities and abide by all state and federal laws and regulations. For the purposes of this text, the authors are addressing typical elements and expectations of an HDS employee or IC.

FINDING EMPLOYMENT

The first step in job hunting is ensuring that you have the right attitude and outlook. It is important to stay positive but also to maintain realistic expectations. You will enhance your chances of finding employment sooner by resourcing yourself well—through networking opportunities, becoming credentialed, and so on—and by following the tips and suggestions in the following sections. Refer back to the Credentialing section of Chapter 1 as needed.

Employee Versus Independent Contractor

An employee works for a hospital or MTSO, either full-time or part-time, and may receive benefits such as paid time off (PTO), holiday pay, sick pay, 401(k), and so on. Employees may work onsite, at home, or a combination of both. Employees may have a set schedule each week, or their hours may vary depending on the workload. In most cases, employees are required to work at least one day on the weekend, or some companies rotate the weekends that their employees are required to work.

An IC is a business owner. An IC is self-employed and receives no benefits from the company or MTSO with which he or she is contracted. The IC must file his or her own taxes, be well versed in proper policies and procedures, comply with other business regulations such as business associate agreements, submit invoices for transcription or editing services, find and pay for his or her own insurance, and so on. The IC might work at home or rent office space. Those who enjoy being on their own and having a flexible schedule will benefit from being an IC.

There is no right or wrong answer for being an employee versus an IC; it is simply what works best for your personality and lifestyle.

Tips for Job Searching and Interviewing

These tips and resources will help enhance your knowledge of the industry and better prepare you for working in the healthcare documentation profession.

- **Become credentialed.** Check out the AHDI website for information about the field of healthcare documentation, AHDI as the professional association for HDSs, and credentialing. Becoming credentialed as a Registered Healthcare Documentation Specialist (RHDS) or a Certified Healthcare Documentation Specialist (CHDS) shows professionalism and respect for your chosen career field and is an external indicator to others of your commitment to the profession and to continuing education. Membership and participation in AHDI will allow you to meet, network with, and make friends with other professionals in the field, learn the latest industry news and trends, and provide job opportunities you otherwise would not have known about. Network! AHDI has local, state, and regional components throughout the United States and Canada. Visit the AHDI website to learn where the nearest AHDI component is and how you can get involved.

- **Update your résumé.** (Read "Tips on Creating an Effective Résumé," p. 15.) You can also go to the AHDI website and type "How to Write a Résumé" in the search box. You will find articles that will offer suggestions for creating an effective résumé. (See p. 17 for a sample.)

- **Create business cards—a true mark of professionalism.** Design and print your own business cards or order them from any number of local or online printing companies. Shop around and look at samples. A simple but professional business card will catch people's eye.

- **Find a mentor.** Some students are fortunate to have the opportunity of an internship or externship with an MTSO before graduation to gain hands-on experience. Others begin their careers as an apprentice with an IC, a person with an at-home business, who is willing to help them get started. For the IC or MTSO, hiring a beginning HDS is both costly and time consuming. New HDSs should be prepared to commit to the job and to learn all they can about creating, transcribing, and editing medical documents as well as how to run a business. New employees can also learn a great deal by working in-house, having access to patient charts, seeing how office personnel work together, and learning how healthcare documentation fits into the larger scheme of things.

- **Explore employment opportunities.** With copies of your résumé and business cards in hand, go to medical office buildings, including pathology laboratories and radiology offices; ask to speak to the office manager. Make an appointment, if necessary. Also search job sites on the Internet. Network with others in the industry to find out which companies are hiring. When you do get an interview, remember to research the company and learn all you can about it so that you can customize your interview answers as to why you want to work for that specific company. An employer is more likely to hire someone who has taken the initiative to learn about his or her company and who also shows enthusiasm and genuine interest in working for the company.

- **Build your network.** Wherever you apply, be sure to pick up that company's business card and keep notes about who you spoke with, including if they are currently hiring or not, whether or not you got an interview, the number of years of experience required, and any other helpful details.

- **Negotiate your worth.** At the interview they are going to want to know what you can offer *them*. Do not be demanding. Instead, be prepared to match your skills to their needs. Make sure they know all your best qualities, how you will fit into their business, and how your expertise will help to make them more successful. Ask that they keep your résumé and business card on file for future reference.

- **Be versatile.** Offer to be backup for the office, covering healthcare documentation or editing for weekends, holidays, sick leave, or vacation time. Offer to help clear up their backlog of work. Getting something to list on your résumé is the most important thing right now.

- **Mind your manners.** When leaving the interview, be gracious, smile, and thank the office manager, the receptionist, and so on, even if they have said "no" to you. Every interview is a learning experience. *Always* write a short, positive thank-you note to your interviewer in your own handwriting. (See the example on page 20.)

- **Think positively.** This whole process is a learning experience. Keep notes so you can evaluate your experience later. Who knows, this may be the first day of the REST OF YOUR LIFE!

Dos and Don'ts Checklist

Being interviewed can be a nerve-wracking process. To help set your mind at ease and be better prepared for your interview, follow the recommendations below provided by experienced interviewers and you are sure to make a positive first impression. *N.B.*: A large percent of the healthcare documentation workforce works from a remote location (e.g., home office). Be prepared to interview by phone or online via Skype or some other technical venue.

☐ DO shake hands with a firm grip, use good eye contact, and smile.

☐ DO use courteous greetings and polite small talk (stay away from controversial topics such as politics and religion).

☐ DO dress professionally and groom neatly, including clean, pressed clothes and shined shoes (no flip-flops, facial piercings, tattoos showing, or low-seated pants).

☐ DO NOT chew gum.

☐ DO keep your cell phone or other electronics on vibrate or turned off.

☐ DO ensure your voice mail phone message is clear and friendly. For example, "I'm away from the phone. Please leave your name and number so I can return your call."

☐ DO NOT bring family members, including children, or friends to your interview. If a family member or friend gave you a ride to your interview, ask him or her to stay in the car or wait in a nearby restaurant.

☐ DO research the company with which you are interviewing. Know pertinent details such as how long they have been in business, whether they have a national presence, and so on, which may come up during the interview.

☐ DO ask questions—make sure they are pertinent to the job for which you are applying. For example, how many HDSs do they employ, do they reimburse or compensate the cost of credentialing exams or continuing education credits, what is the supervisory structure, do they use QA personnel and give feedback on errors found, and so on.

☐ DO prepare a brief introductory speech about yourself—who you are, what your background is, what you are looking for, and why you are perfect for this job—two to three minutes tops.

☐ DO follow up the interview with a personal thank-you note. (See the sample on page 20.)

☐ DO contact the interviewer about three days after the interview to let him or her know how much you appreciate the meeting, how much you would like to work at the company, and so on. Be ready for follow-up questions and a potential second interview. A second interview may be with someone else—someone higher up in the company—so stay prepared.

See Appendix G for more resources on interviewing.

Tips for Creating an Effective Résumé

Your résumé is often the first opportunity a potential employer has to learn about you. It presents a snapshot of your work experience and education. It is a timeline intended to catch an employer's eye and show what you can do for the company; therefore, it should stand apart from other résumés the employer might have received. Although the document gives a picture of you, it should be short and to the point.

In creating a résumé, here are some pointers:

Begin with your *personal contact information*: Insert your complete legal name, address, phone numbers, fax number, and email address as the heading for the page.

Next list your *employment objective:* This statement should be concise but reflect thought. It should include more than just what you *want*; it should include what you can *offer*. Use different objective statements for different jobs. You can have more than one résumé.

In the next section, describe your *educational background,** with the most recent educational experience listed first, such as the certificate you may have just earned. Any extra classes you completed should be listed, too (e.g., electronic health records, coding and billing).

List your *work experience*, with the most recent job first. For each job, list the dates employed (month and year), employer's name, job title, supervisor, contact number, and your primary responsibilities. When you list your duties, use action verbs (e.g., answered phones, filed medical records, and confirmed appointments). Also, be sure that the statements are parallel in grammatical structure.

Because this section of the résumé is a timeline, if there was a time you were not working,

---

*These educational background and work experience sections can be reversed depending on what information is most pertinent to the job for which you are applying.

indicate what you were doing (e.g., out of town assisting a relative, touring Europe, recovering from surgery). Include any part-time or summer jobs or volunteer projects that show you are responsible and dependable and that you would be an asset.

List any experience you had with medical transcription platforms such as DocuScribe or DocuManage.

If you worked two jobs at one time, be sure to include the days of the week or the shifts so that it is easy to see how they meshed together. For example, maybe you do one thing during the week and something else on weekends. You might have a full-time day job with a part-time evening job. However, if your part-time job is not pertinent to either your experience or the career field in which you are interested, you can leave it out.

In the next section, include areas of interest, hobbies, school or community activities, and participation in service organizations. Include special skills, such as being bilingual, knowing sign language, knowing cardiopulmonary resuscitation, and so on.

A comment about references should be the last line of the résumé. You can simply write, "References available upon request." Information relative to references should be listed on a separate page and carried to the interview—it is given to the interviewer only upon request.

Ask someone else to proofread your résumé for accuracy. A huge part of being an HDS is accuracy, so make sure it is reflected in your résumé.

Remember, this is the only picture of you that the prospective employer has. The ideal résumé is one page long, but two pages can be acceptable.

REMEMBER: Your résumé must stand out from the crowd! Employers throw résumés with typos into the trash!

(Sample Résumé)

Phoenix Lee Sharp
140 Chapel Road #9A
Athens, GA 30605
706.555.5501 (cell)
plsharprn@yahoo.com

OBJECTIVE   To work as a human resources manager in a multi-physician clinic

EDUCATION   Florida State University, Tallahassee, FL: BS in Nursing with minor in Human Resources Management, Aug 2003

Miami-Dade Community College, Miami, FL: AA degree in Anatomy & Physiology, May 1998

EXPERIENCE   Dec 2004 to Present **The Nashville Diagnostic Clinic**
Title: RN

Duties: Assist physicians with patient care, help in minor surgical procedures, keep instruments sterile, help in dictation of reports, maintain employees' HIPAA and CPR status, and other office duties as required.

Supervisor: Fred Anderson, MD, Phone: 615.901.1111 ext 35

Dec 1998 to Nov 2004 **James C. Thompson Memorial Clinic**
Title: Human Resource Assistant

Duties: Assisted HR director with day-to-day activities of the department, communicated with personnel relative to individual employment issues, and conducted new employee orientation and training.

Supervisor: Kenneth Williams, Director, Phone: 731.555.3700 ext 90

Aug 1995 to Dec 1998 **Forrest General Medical Center**
Title: RN

Duties: Assisted with hospital patient care; supervised surgical floor nursing duties, worked various shifts, maintained employees' HIPAA and CPR status, organized nursing shifts, and filled in when necessary.

Supervisor: Tyron Nguyen, RN, Phone: 615.555.5000 ext. 72

HONORS   **Florida State University**
Outstanding senior nursing major, president of Student Nursing
Association, and vice president of Student Human Resources
Association

Miami-Dade Community College
Beta Club, student government association, and yearbook staff

REFERENCES AVAILABLE UPON REQUEST
(*N.B.*: References should be typed on a separate page and taken
to the interview. Provide each reference's full legal name, position,
address, phone number, and email address.)

REFERENCE EXAMPLE (submitted separately upon request)

Kenneth Williams, Director
Human Resources Department
James C. Thompson Memorial Clinic
#1 Lincoln Circle
Paris, TN 37904
Phone: 731.555.3700 ext 90
k.williams@yahoo.com

Sample Cover Letter (to accompany résumé)

Phoenix Lee Sharp
140 Chapel Road #9A
Athens, GA 30605
706.555.5501 (cell)
plsharprn@yahoo.com

Fred Anderson, MD
The Nashville Diagnostic Clinic
12221 N. Cleary Expressway
Nashville, TN 37758

Dear Dr. Anderson:

Ms. Charlotte Patterson, a nurse employed at the clinic, referred me for a job as manager of Human Resources at The Nashville Diagnostic Clinic. I have several years' experience working as a clinic nurse, including working in human resources, which should qualify me for this job.

Please review the enclosed résumé for additional information about my education and related work experience. I am available for an interview at your convenience.

Thank you for your consideration.

(handwritten signature here)

Enclosure

(Sample Thank-You Letter)

Phoenix Lee Sharp
140 Chapel Road #9A
Athens, GA 30605
706.555.5501 (cell)
plsharp@yahoo.com

July 28, ----

Fred Anderson, MD
The Nashville Diagnostic Clinic
12221 N. Cleary Expressway
Nashville, TN 37758

Dear Dr. Anderson:

I would like to express my thanks for the time you spent with me yesterday for both the interview and the tour of your facilities. It is clear that you have devoted yourself to providing the best in clinical and diagnostic care for your patients.

I look forward to hearing from you in the near future.

Most sincerely,

(add handwritten signature here)

N.B.: The handwritten thank-you note is part of the etiquette used when looking for a job; it is an important part of the process.

Computer Best Practices

Employees are expected to keep their computers and workstations neat and sanitary. After all, employees often share workstations. If a computer malfunction occurs, the IT department can be called for repair. An IC is responsible for all the business's computers and equipment—onsite and offsite. It could be a sound decision to contract with a company to keep the computers running well with files backed up on a nightly basis. Maintaining patient computer files is a vital part of an IC's job.

Employees and ICs alike use computer passwords, and these can be problematic. Obviously, each person's password is private; however, our passwords are supposed to be difficult to access. The most effective passwords are those that use the most variety of characters. The problem is how to remember it. We write them on Post-it Notes and stick them all around, making "privacy" null and void. With the global onslaught of computer hacking, we all need a better plan to safeguard medical records. This could be a potential liability issue, especially for ICs. A number of free and paid applications, or "apps," are available to download on a computer, smart phone, or other mobile device that can be used to store and manage any variety of work and personal passwords in a secure manner.

Another sound decision is to never forward random emails to people on your contact list. It makes you look unprofessional at best, ultimately hurting your career; at worst, it can cause people to block your correspondence. Never use a company's email account to send emails to personal contacts. People can mark such emails as spam, which could result in your company's email server being put on a black list as a spammer.

Certain things are appropriate to forward; for example, the latest industry news is relevant to a list of people to whom it will matter. These shared tidbits are important for keeping current in your career. Forward select association news to those whom you know would be interested. Forward positive information regarding your company. Everyone likes to see their company gain positive exposure. Essentially, forward purposeful news that is relevant to the receivers.

Keep in mind, however, that some people will not be interested in even this type of forwarding. Include a brief note in your email explaining why you forwarded the email (e.g., continuing education opportunity, important drug updates included, new terms list) and include an invitation for recipients to be removed from your "forwarded emails" list if they so desire. Respect their requests by remembering to remove them from the list of people to whom you forward emails.

CONTINUING EDUCATION AND CAREER ADVANCEMENT

Just as important as the building blocks are in obtaining a good education, so too is continuing education in staying current with the latest terminology, treatments, studies, equipment, and other tools of the trade. As an employee, staying up with the newest trends in your field is not only personally valuable but also a good way to advance in your career. As an IC, staying current is essential for business. It is also important to provide educational opportunities for any subcontractors you may have.

As has been mentioned previously, AHDI offers continuing education online at every level for HDSs and students. The Internet is a fountain of continuing education possibilities, including free Web videos. Taking advantage of local, state, regional, and national AHDI meetings and conferences offers credentialed HDS practitioners and students the chance to attend presentations online and in person. It offers organizational, travel, networking, and volunteer opportunities.

It is no longer possible or even advisable to stay in one position throughout an entire career. Education today leads people onward and upward, especially in the field of medicine. With research bringing us new treatments, medications, and equipment every year, no one can afford to remain static and immobile. We all must consider ourselves continual learners in today's world. One of the best things about being an HDS is that no matter how long you are in this business, you never stop learning.

UNIT 2

LISTENING SKILLS:
DO YOU HEAR WHAT I HEAR?

CHAPTER 3

DECIPHERING ACCENTS

KEY TERMS

cleft palate
diphthong
English as a second language (ESL)
intonation
lisp

phonetics
rhythm
stress
stuttering
vocal polyps or nodules

LEARNING OBJECTIVES

1. Assess your temperament for English-as-a-second-language (ESL) speakers.
2. Identify the components that make up an accent.
3. Learn to differentiate sounds and syllables.
4. Understand how to assess dictation appropriateness for inclusion in the record.

INTRODUCTION

For many healthcare documentation specialists (HDSs), deciphering accented dictation can be difficult at best; downright frustrating and seemingly impossible at worst. By training our ears to the various nuances of speech patterns, we can perfect our craft, thus making the HDS more valuable. This includes regional accents, foreign accents, and certain speech disorders (**lisps**, **stuttering**, and **cleft palate**). Even long-time smokers may exhibit dictation fluctuations caused by **vocal polyps** or **nodules**.

Whether you are a new HDS or one who has been transcribing or editing for years, the first thing of which to take notice and evaluate is the attitude and temperament you embody at work. Are you becoming frustrated or irritable every time a difficult dictator comes up in the queue? Or perhaps only those who give you the most trouble bring up negative emotions. How fast a dictator speaks will play a major part in how well you understand what is being spoken. Embrace the challenge of learning and understanding difficult and accented dictation. Learning medical terminology is similar to learning a foreign language, so you are now learning to hear words you already know—a "language" you have already conquered—with a different em-PHA-sis.

A person's accent is based on pronunciation. Pronunciation of words is usually learned based on a person's surroundings: a particular location and those with whom the person is in frequent contact (including home, school, and social settings). **Phonetics** is "the study of speech sounds, their production and combination, and their representation by certain symbols." The International Phonetic Alphabet is "an alphabet for international use, designed to represent each human speech sound by a single symbol" (Webster's, 2002). In any language, the components that make up an accent include intonation, rhythm, stress, and, of course, vowels and consonants.

COMPONENTS OF AN ACCENT

In the American English language, vowels include A, E, I, O, U, and sometimes Y. Vowel sounds are made by using the vocal cords. These few letters make up approximately 20 sounds in most American English accents, thus contributing to pronunciation difficulties of many **English as a second language (ESL)** learners. Table 3-1 lists the symbols for vowel sounds and corresponding word examples.

Consonants make up the rest of the letters of the American English alphabet: B, C, D, F, G, H, J, K, L, M, N, R, S, T, V, W, X, Y, and Z. When a consonant is spoken, air is partially blocked as the sound is made, creating a less clear sound than when vowels are spoken and drawing out the length of the sound. Table 3-2 lists the symbols for consonant sounds and corresponding word examples.

Intonation is the "pitch" pattern of speech, the rise and fall of the voice as one speaks. A voice can be pitched high, as in the soprano singing voice, or low, as in the baritone singing voice. In English, typically the voice is pitched down at the end of a declarative sentence. When we ask a question, the voice typically is pitched higher at the end.

How fast or slow a person speaks is called **rhythm**. It can change from person to person and from language to language.

When talking about **stress** in language, this refers to sounds and syllables that are spoken harder or longer. Stress patterns differ in various languages; therefore, emphasis on different parts of a word as spoken by an ESL dictator versus an American English speaker is often heard. For example, the word *tinnitus* may be pronounced with the stress or emphasis on the

TABLE 3-1 SYMBOLS FOR VOWEL SOUNDS

Symbol	Key Words
A	at, cap, parrot
Ā	ape, play, sail
Ä	cot, father, heart
E	ten, wealth, merry
Ē	even, feet, money
I	is, stick, mirror
Ī	ice, high, sky
Ō	go, open, tone
Ô	all, lawn, horn
Oo	could, look, pull
Yoo	cure, furious, your
Ōō	boot, crew, tune
Yōō	cute, few, use
Oi	boy, oil, royal
Ou	cow, out, sour
U	mud, ton, blood, trouble
ʊ	her, sir, word
ə	ago, agent, collect, focus
'	cattle, paddle, sudden, sweeten

TABLE 3-2 SYMBOLS FOR CONSONANT SOUNDS

Symbol	Key Words
B	bed, table, rob
D	dog, middle, sad
F	for, phone, cough
G	get, wiggle, dog
H	hat, hope, ahead
Hw	which, white
J	joy, badge, agent
K	kill, cat, quiet
L	let, yellow, ball
M	meet, number, time
N	net, candle, ton
P	put, sample, escape
R	red, wrong, born
S	sit, castle, office
T	top, letter, cat
V	voice, every, love
W	wet, always, quart
Y	yes, canyon, onion
Z	zoo, misery, rise
Ch	chew, nature, punch
Sh	shell, machine, bush
Th	thin, nothing, truth
Th	then, other, bathe
Zh	beige, measure, seizure
Ŋ	ring, anger, drink

middle syllable ("tin-NI-tus") or on the beginning syllable ("TIN-ni-tus").

The HDS must also be aware of sounds spoken that are not actual words. A dictator may start to speak but get sidetracked or change his or her mind about what he or she was going to say, with the speech trailing off. Likewise, a dictator may hem haw at the end of a sentence, inserting an "um" or "uh," mumble, or speak an aside to a colleague. A phrase often spoken but that can wreak havoc is "period paragraph." Heavily accented, this phrase can be difficult to understand. Dictators often insert words related to punctuation, where they think it should go (whether correct or not); the HDS can confuse this with verbiage to be entered into the patient's record. ESL dictators tend to repeat their words and paragraphs in each report. After the accented dictators' styles have been learned, the HDS can get through this work with no problems and may eventually be considered an "expert" in accented dictation.

ACCENTS PRONOUNCED

In accented dictation, a simple "thank you" can sound like "tanks" or "sank you" for those who cannot pronounce a **diphthong** (th). "Please" can sound like "peas" or "peace" when the "l" or the "s" cannot be pronounced. The "bl" and "br" sounds can be hard to pronounce in some languages; in others, the "r" and "l" sounds can be interchanged, as can "v" and "w" sounds. See the following examples of how accented dictation may sound (Table 3-3).

Also, be aware of language in its global sense. A word such as "loo," which means "bathroom" in England, is well known throughout the world.

USING GOOD JUDGMENT

People, physicians included, can get away with much more in the spoken word than in the written word. That is one reason transcriptionists are vital. We have the innate ability to know the difference. The spoken word is more relaxed and spontaneous, and the written word is more formal by its very nature—certainly in the medical record.

The phrase, "no barriers to communication" has been dictated in countless medical reports, usually when the patient's primary language is not English. Often, a relative is present to translate for the patient. This phrase reinforces the patient's understanding of what the physician is explaining and that there are no issues with

TABLE 3-3 COMMON WORDS IDENTIFIED IN ACCENTED DICTATION

Common Word	Sound in Accented Dictation
blood	bud
breathe	bleathe or bleed
BUN	bun (pronounced as a word)
ear	eh or eah
Jell-O	yellow
neoplasm	leoplas (with no final m)
present	pwesent
relief	le-eef or reweef
there, their	dere
they're	the-uh
think	tink or sink
this	dis or zis
these	dees or zees
thought	taut
thyroid	ti-roid
values	falues
very	werry
viral	wiral
VSD	wee-es-dee
VY-plasty	wee-wi plasty
water	vater or vata

miscommunication. It is also required for legal purposes—liability.

Other phrases often found at the end of a patient's report include "dictated but not read"; "signed but not read"; and "dictated but not read, subject to transcription variation." Physicians are busy and sometimes use this rubber-stamped disclaimer, thinking it excuses them from errors or omissions on reports or correspondence they sign. However, such statements may actually increase liability. If an unreviewed report contains an error that results in patient injury, the patient could allege that the doctor was "too busy" or "not concerned enough" to ensure the accuracy of their medical record.

What does "transcription variation" mean? In this context, transcription variation may be any liberties an HDS may have taken while editing a report that varies from what was dictated. It is necessary to document patient care, but many clinicians do not particularly enjoy it. Although most do their best to dictate concisely and accurately, clinicians are usually more focused on providing good patient care than making sure they dotted all the I's and crossed all the T's while dictating. HDSs are trained to listen for and correct such things as grammatical errors, subject-verb agreement, spelling, punctuation placement, correct use of pronouns, and rewording of a statement or phrase for clarity of intended meaning. This is not to suggest that an HDS should rewrite or tamper with what is dictated simply to make it sound better but should only reword when absolutely needed so that the statement or phrase will not be misinterpreted. Remember, the medical meaning should never be altered.

Example:

D: I told the patient to take the 10 oxy dispensed for pain every 6 hours.

T: I told the patient to take the oxycodone, 10 dispensed, for pain every 6 hours.

~or~

T: I told the patient to take the oxycodone (10 dispensed) for pain every 6 hours.

The HDS should always check and follow facility and client guidelines for editing preferences and policies.

Transcription variation may also occur when the dictator has made inappropriate comments or used bad language, has criticized another health professional, or refers to patients using racial or religious slurs. Such negative statements should not be included in a patient's medical record. The HDS must be able to know when the dictator is venting, joking, or just being rude. The HDS should follow appropriate facility or client policies and guidelines when a similar occurrence is encountered. When in doubt, elevate the report to a supervisor or manager to take appropriate action.

If a potential legal issue or complaint is mentioned by the dictator (e.g., complaining about the nursing staff or an inappropriate action by another clinician—something that does not necessarily pertain to the patient), follow appropriate facility or client policies and guidelines or submit it to the supervisor or the office manager so it can be pursued.

You will find more resources about accents in Appendix G.

CHAPTER 4

MEDICATIONS: USAGE, IDIOSYNCRASIES, AND SOUND-ALIKES

KEY TERMS

intramuscular
intrathecal
mnemonics

sublingual
transdermal

LEARNING OBJECTIVES

1. Examine why correct medication and dosage identification is critical.
2. Name the various routes and methods of administering medications.

3. Classify medications by type and give examples.

INTRODUCTION

When editing medical reports, emphasis is placed on spelling, punctuation, and grammar issues. These are all important, but the dictation of drugs, their dosages, and routes of administration are critical to patient care.

USAGE

Numerous new prescription and over-the-counter medications and supplements come on the market each year. It is of utmost importance that healthcare documentation specialists stay up to date on the latest pharmacologic releases in order to accurately and efficiently identify the correct medications and dosages being listed in a speech-recognized document in addition to any dictated errors.

The best way to prevent errors in dictated or transcribed medication usage is to avoid abbreviations. Go to http://www.medabbrev.com and click on "Controlled Vocabulary" to read about the dangers of abbreviations in health care. Consider "DT"—we know this abbreviation to mean delirium tremens. However, a search of the website shows that DT has 15 other possible meanings. Even "TV" has 15 possible meanings on the website. It is clear that even the simplest abbreviations can be misread, misconstrued, and mistaken.

The healthcare documentation specialist (HDS) should know and be able to identify:

- The correct spelling of a medication.
- Dosages in which the medication is given (adult and pediatric).
- The route in which the medication is administered (oral, **transdermal**, intravenous injection, **sublingual**, rectal, **intrathecal**, **intramuscular**, and so on). (See Table 4-1.)
- What the medication is used for or the conditions being treated.

TABLE 4-1 ROUTES OF MEDICATION ADMINISTRATION

ROUTE	METHOD OF ADMINISTRATION
Oral	**Having patient swallow drug**
Enteral route	Administer through a tube
Sublingual	Place drug under the tongue
Buccal	Place drug between cheek and gum
Parenteral	**Injecting drug into**
Subcutaneous injection	Subcutaneous tissue
Intramuscular injection	Muscle tissue
Intradermal injection	Subepidermis
Intravenous injection	Vein
Intraarterial injection	Artery
Intracardiac injection	Heart tissue
Intraperitoneal injection	Peritoneal cavity
Intraspinal injection	Spinal canal
Intraosseous injection	Bone
Topical	**Inserting drug into**
Vaginal administration	Vagina
Rectal administration	Rectum
Inunction	Skin via rubbing
Instillation	Mucous membrane via direct contact
Irrigation	Mucous membrane via drug solution
Skin application	Skin via transdermal patch
Pulmonary	**Inhalation of drug**

Source: Stedman's Medical Dictionary

HDSs are expected to be aware of the facts surrounding the dictation of medications and should always be asking, "Does the medication and dosage dictated make sense in the context of the document?" There is absolutely no guessing allowed. If you are not certain, visit reputable Internet sites or use your pharmaceutical drug book to research it. Drug books should be updated every year or two. (See Appendix G.)

IDIOSYNCRASIES

Medication names can be long, can sound similar to another word, and may have tricky spelling. The ability to decipher the correct medication intended and its spelling is made more complex based on various correct and incorrect pronunciations, an originator's accent, an HDS's knowledge base of medications and their uses, and of course the dictation of the correct word intended.

Not all printed drug books on the market include pronunciation indicators, so an educated guess based on rules of the English language is sometimes the best we can hope for. However, our ever-advancing world of technology not only provides an array of electronic resources at our fingertips but also allows us to go beyond the basics. A drug manufacturer's website may or may not provide drug pronunciation, but many sites dedicated to drug and prescription medication information do. In fact, sites such as www .drugs.com not only include the pronunciation key but also have audio pronunciations available. (See Appendix G.)

A person's accent (Southern United States, Asian, Latin, Canadian, Eastern Indian, and so on) will also affect pronunciation. Emphasis on certain syllables, extra syllables, or the rhythm of a native language can often make it more challenging for an HDS to decode and reveal the words behind the accent. More information about this topic can be found in Chapter 3: Deciphering Accents.

Naturally good spellers will have a great advantage over poor spellers in this area. Some **mnemonics** learned as a child, such as "I before E except after C," stick with us and come naturally as we pen (or transcribe) medical language. The language of medicine, however, based largely on ancient Latin and Greek, seems to have rules of its own.

A NOTE ABOUT LANGUAGES . . .

Romance languages are those developed from Latin and include Italian, French, and Spanish. Germanic languages comprise a branch of the Indo-European language family containing English, German, Dutch, Afrikaans, and the Scandinavian languages. The Celtic language is spoken in Ireland, Scotland, the Isle of Man, Wales, Cornwall, and Brittany. Greek, a Hellenic language, is unique to Greece.

The language heard on dictation for this text is American English. Our foreign physicians have accents, but they dictate in American English. This includes all the peccadilloes we use in this country, region by region. Those from the Northeast, the Midwest, the South, and the West use regional phrases in dictation. Ever heard of "stovepipe legs"? It is a condition of massive obesity that simulates lymphedema. When it involves both legs, it is referred to as "stovepipe legs" in the South. Some clinicians dictate "zero" or "none" as "nil" or "aught." In New England, a milkshake is called a "frappe." Regional words and phrases will come up in dictation, and as well-trained medical editors, we must be prepared to edit them correctly.

In the manufacturing process, medication names are created based on stems, which connect to a particular drug class or mode of action. By figuring out what a stem means, you can likely figure out what a drug does. For example, the stem -*prazol* means the drug is a benzimidazole antiulcer agent. Therefore, drugs containing that stem (e.g., omeprazole, lansoprazole, and pantoprazole) can be readily identified as belonging to a group of drugs called proton pump inhibitors, which decrease the amount of acid in the stomach. (See Table 4-2.) Word association is paramount to an HDS's understanding and recognition of both existing and future-named medication. By breaking down the components within a word to determine the meaning and memorizing these patterns in medication names, an HDS's knowledge is enhanced, and the job of medical editing becomes much easier.

SOUND-ALIKES

Medication names can sound similar. Likewise, numbers can sound similar when dosage information is being dictated. Therefore, it is imperative for HDSs to use their knowledge of medications and dosages to apply critical thinking skills as they listen along with voice files. HDSs should keep surrounding report context in mind, such as past medical history, to include conditions, symptoms, and disease processes, the patient's age, and diagnoses. Knowing such pieces of information makes it that much easier to correctly identify an unclear-sounding drug (and its dosage) while listening to dictation.

A robust list of general medications can be found in Appendix C, but Table 4-3 lists a sampling of common medications that sound alike and may easily be confused with other medications or other medical words heard in transcription and editing.

TABLE 4-2 GENERIC MEDICATION STEMS, CATEGORIES, AND EXAMPLES

Stems apply only to generic names.

Stems	Drug Class or Drug Category	Examples (Generic Names)
-afil	Phosphodiesterase (PDE) inhibitors	sildenafil, tadalafil, vardenafil
-asone	Corticosteroids	betamethasone, dexamethasone, diflorasone, fluticasone, mometasone
-bicin	Antineoplastic, cytotoxic agents	doxorubicin, epirubicin, idarubicin, valrubicin
-bital	Barbiturates (sedatives)	butabarbital, butalbital, phenobarbital, secobarbital
-caine	Local anesthetics	bupivacaine, lidocaine, mepivacaine, prilocaine, proparacaine
cef-, ceph-	Cephalosporin antibiotics	cefaclor, cefdinir, cefixime, cefprozil, cephalexin
-cillin	Penicillin antibiotics	amoxicillin, ampicillin, dicloxacillin, nafcillin, oxacillin
Cort	Corticosteroids	clocortolone, fludrocortisone, hydrocortisone
-cycline	Tetracycline antibiotics	demeclocycline, doxycycline, minocycline, tetracycline
-dazole	Anthelmintics, antibiotics, antibacterials	albendazole, mebendazole, metronidazole, tinidazole
-dipine	Calcium channel blockers	amlodipine, felodipine, nifedipine, nimodipine, nisoldipine
-dronate	Bisphosphonates, bone resorption inhibitors	alendronate, etidronate, ibandronate, risedronate
-eprazole	Proton pump inhibitors	esomeprazole, omeprazole, rabeprazole
-fenac	Nonsteroidal antiinflammatory drugs	bromfenac, diclofenac, nepafenac
-floxacin	Quinolone antibiotics	besifloxacin, ciprofloxacin, levofloxacin, moxifloxacin, ofloxacin
-gliptin	Antidiabetics, inhibitors of the DPP-4 enzyme	saxagliptin, sitagliptin, linagliptin
-glitazone	Antidiabetics, thiazolidinediones	pioglitazone, rosiglitazone, troglitazone
-iramine	Antihistamines	brompheniramine, chlorpheniramine, pheniramine
-lamide	Carbonic anhydrase inhibitors	acetazolamide, brinzolamide, dorzolamide, methazolamide
-mab	Monoclonal antibodies	adalimumab, daclizumab, infliximab, omalizumab, trastuzumab
-mustine	Alkylating agents (antineoplastics)	carmustine, estramustine, lomustine, bendamustine
-mycin	Antibiotics, antibacterials	azithromycin, clarithromycin, clindamycin, erythromycin
-nacin	Muscarinic antagonists (anticholinergics)	darifenacin, solifenacin
-nazole	Antifungals	fluconazole, ketoconazole, miconazole, terconazole
-olol	Beta-blockers	atenolol, metoprolol, nadolol, pindolol, propranolol, timolol
-olone	Corticosteroids	fluocinolone, fluorometholone, prednisolone, triamcinolone
-olone	Anabolic steroids	nandrolone, oxandrolone, oxymetholone
-onide	Corticosteroids	budesonide, ciclesonide, desonide, fluocinonide, halcinonide
-oprazole	Proton pump inhibitors	dexlansoprazole, lansoprazole, pantoprazole
parin, -parin	Antithrombotics, anticoagulants (blood thinners)	dalteparin, enoxaparin, fondaparinux, heparin, tinzaparin

TABLE 4-2 (CONTINUED)

-phylline	Xanthine derivatives (bronchodilators)	aminophylline, dyphylline, oxtriphylline, theophylline
-pramine	Tricyclic antidepressants	clomipramine, desipramine, imipramine, trimipramine
pred, pred-	Corticosteroids	loteprednol, prednicarbate, prednisolone, prednisone
-pril	Angiotensin-converting enzyme inhibitors	benazepril, captopril, enalapril, lisinopril, moexipril, ramipril
-profen	Nonsteroidal antiinflammatory drugs	fenoprofen, flurbiprofen, ibuprofen, ketoprofen
-ridone	Atypical antipsychotics	iloperidone, paliperidone, risperidone
-sartan	Angiotensin II receptor antagonists	candesartan, irbesartan, losartan, olmesartan, valsartan
-semide	Loop diuretics (water pills)	furosemide, torsemide
-setron	Serotonin 5-HT3 receptor antagonists	alosetron, dolasetron, granisetron, ondansetron, palonosetron
-setron	Antiemetics and antinauseants	dolasetron, granisetron, ondansetron, palonosetron
-statin	HMG-CoA reductase inhibitors, statins	atorvastatin, lovastatin, pitavastatin, pravastatin, rosuvastatin, simvastatin
sulfa-	Antibiotics, antiinfectives, antiinflammatories	sulfacetamide, sulfadiazine, sulfamethoxazole, sulfasalazine
-tadine	Antihistamines	cyproheptadine, desloratadine, loratadine, olopatadine
-tadine	Antivirals, anti-influenza-A agents	amantadine, rimantadine
-terol	Beta-agonists, bronchodilators	albuterol, arformoterol, formoterol, levalbuterol, salmeterol
-thiazide	Thiazide diuretics (water pills)	chlorothiazide, hydrochlorothiazide, methyclothiazide
-tinib	Antineoplastics (kinase inhibitors)	crizotinib, dasatinib, erlotinib, gefitinib, imatinib
-trel	Female hormones (progestins)	desogestrel, etonogestrel, levonorgestrel, norgestrel
tretin-, tretin, -tretin	Retinoids, dermatologic agents, forms of vitamin A	acitretin, alitretinoin, isotretinoin, tretinoin
-triptan	Antimigraines, selective 5-HT receptor agonists	almotriptan, eletriptan, rizatriptan, sumatriptan, zolmitriptan
-tyline	Tricyclic antidepressants	amitriptyline, nortriptyline, protriptyline
vir, -vir	Antivirals, anti-HIV agents	abacavir, efavirenz, enfuvirtide, nevirapine, ritonavir, tenofovir
vir, -vir	Antivirals, anti-hepatitis agents	adefovir, entecavir, ribavirin (along with interferon)
-vir	Antivirals, anti-herpes agents	acyclovir, famciclovir, penciclovir, valacyclovir
-vir	Antivirals, anti-cytomegalovirus agents	cidofovir, ganciclovir, valganciclovir
-vir	Antivirals, anti-flu agents	oseltamivir, zanamivir
-vudine	Antivirals, nucleoside analogues	lamivudine, stavudine, telbivudine, zidovudine
-zepam	Benzodiazepines	clonazepam, diazepam, flurazepam, lorazepam, temazepam
-zodone	Antidepressants	nefazodone, trazodone, vilazodone
-zolam	Benzodiazepines	alprazolam, estazolam, midazolam, triazolam
-zosin	Alpha blockers	alfuzosin, doxazosin, prazosin, terazosin

Source: U.S. Food and Drug Administration

TABLE 4-3 COMMON MEDICATION SOUND-ALIKES

Medication	Sound-alike
Aciphex	AcuTect
Actonel	Atenolol
Afrin	Aspirin
Allergan	allergen, Auralgan
Alustra	Lustra
Amaryl	Reminyl
amoxicillin	amoxapine
Anacin	Unisom, Unasyn
Atacand	Ativan
Avita	Evista
Azulfadine	Silvadene
Cardene	Cardizem
Cefzil	Cefadyl, Kefzol
Celexa	Celebrex
Cerebyx	Celebrex
Cidex	Cedax
Cipro	Septa, Septra
clonidine	Klonopin, quinidine
Darvon	Diovan
Decadron	Decaderm, Percodan
digoxin	digitoxin
Dilantin	Mylanta, Xalatan
Enbrel	Limbrel
Femiron	Remeron
fentanyl	Sentinel
Fioricet	Lorcet
Gabitril	Carbatrol

TABLE 4-3 (CONTINUED)

Hycodan	Hycomine, Vicodin
Hytone	Vytone
Isordil	Isuprel
Lasix	Lidex, Esidrix
Lidex	Lasix, Lidox, Wydase
Lincocin	Cleocin, Indocin
Microzide	Maxzide
Narcan	Marcaine
Natacyn	Naprosyn
niacin	Minocin
Nizoral	Nasarel
Orabase	Orinase
oxycodone	OxyContin, Roxicodone
Pamelor	Dymelor, Panlor
Percodan	Decadron
Perdiem	Pyridium
Phenergan	Theragran
Provera	Covera
Restoril	Risperdal, Vistaril, Zestril
Tenex	Xanax
timolol	atenolol
TobraDex	Tobrex
uracil	Uracel, Uracid
Valium	thallium
Xanax	Zantac, Tenex
Zarontin	Zaroxolyn
Zestril	Restoril, Vistaril

Source: Saunders Pharmaceutical Word Book

CHAPTER 5

FRONT-END VERSUS BACK-END SPEECH RECOGNITION

KEY TERMS

back-end speech recognition technology
draft document
flag
front-end speech recognition technology
homonyms
homophones

learned language
negative contractions
real time
speech recognition editor
word salad

LEARNING OBJECTIVES

1. Understand what speech recognition is and the difference between front-end and back-end speech recognition.

2. Name at least three reasons speech recognition is helpful.

3. Identify at least three causes of speech recognition errors.

4. Recite at least three skills required of speech recognition editors.

INTRODUCTION

Speech recognition (SR) is the process of a computer program capturing and converting sounds, words, and phrases into text, with the goal of creating faster and more efficient documentation. SR technology is widely used. SR applications in such devices as smart phones, tablets, and personal computers, and even newer vehicles can be activated to use voice command prompts. In the case of a vehicle, Bluetooth technology can be used to change the radio station, adjust the air conditioning, or dial the phone. This wireless communications system is used with mobile phones, headsets, medical equipment, and more. In the healthcare domain, SR can be implemented in the front end or back end of the medical documentation process.

FRONT-END SPEECH RECOGNITION TECHNOLOGY

Front-end speech recognition technology (SRT) includes such consumer applications as Dragon Naturally Speaking by ScanSoft and Via Voice by IBM. Clinician users of front-end SRT dictate into a personal computer's (PC's) microphone, and the spoken words are then converted to text in a word-processing application in **real time**. This effectively eliminates the need for a transcriptionist to key in the report. For front-end SRT to be as accurate as possible, the user must immediately correct errors made by the software so the program will "learn" the nuances of the user's speech patterns. An SR engine's inability to "learn" speech patterns will perpetuate errors being captured and recorded in medical reports. Only a relatively few clinicians use front-end SRT at this time because it takes considerably longer to use front-end SRT effectively than it does to simply dictate in the traditional manner, but the number of users is steadily increasing. Front-end SRT is better suited for specialties such as radiology, in which terms and phrases of dictated results are highly repetitive. For example, the many types of normal radiography reports can be done via template.

BACK-END SPEECH RECOGNITION TECHNOLOGY

Large institutions and clinics use **back-end speech recognition technology (SRT)**. With this method, the actual speech-to-text conversion takes place *after* the speaker has dictated rather than concurrently. The dictation is recorded in digital form at the time of dictation; and the digital voice files are then processed by a powerful computer running SRT software and converted to a draft text document. A human **speech recognition editor** (healthcare documentation specialist [HDS]) must then listen to the voice file while proofreading the **draft document** because even the most sophisticated SRT applications are not nearly accurate enough to eliminate the need for human review. For example, consider the myriad **homonyms** and **homophones** or the proper placement of punctuation, which creates challenges for a machine that can only translate the speech to text based on how it was programmed—and in some cases, what was dictated. Clinicians often dictate punctuation, but it is not always correctly done.

SPEECH RECOGNITION CHALLENGES

Speech recognition technology has become a preferred method of healthcare documentation by many healthcare facilities. There are some obstacles to overcome, but improvements are continually being made to enhance productivity and efficiency, providing more user-friendly software for SR editors. Numerous healthcare documentation businesses use traditional transcription along with SR in order to offer healthcare facilities more options.

The quality of SR can range from excellent to poor, with whole words and sentences possibly missing from the report. This can happen even with the best dictators. Sometimes **negative contractions**—a negative verb construction that ends in *n't*, such as didn't, won't, and isn't—or the word "not" are dropped. (*N.B.*: Contractions are not allowed in transcribed medical records, even if dictated, regardless of verbatim requirements, except within a direct quote.) Another critical word that may be omitted by SR not interpreting a clinician's speech correctly is "no." The inclusion or omission of "no" can have a huge impact on patient care. For example, an SR engine may erroneously capture "There is *no* pulmonary embolus seen" as "There *is* pulmonary embolus seen." Because of this error, the patient may be provided unnecessary treatment. Additionally, inaccurate information is now in the patient's medical record, perpetuating (1) followup visits, (2) the potential addition of medication the patient needs to take (e.g., an anticoagulant), and (3) financial costs associated with these treatments—all unnecessarily. Insurance and liability will also be impacted.

The beginning of a sentence is another place where "no" is commonly dropped, giving an opposite meaning to the statement made. For example, "No blood transfusion required" is captured as "Blood transfusion required." As stated earlier, this could have a disastrous effect on patient care.

Background noise can also play a part in poor quality output of speech-recognized dictation. These noises may be picked up by the SR engine and translated into something unintelligible. Critical thinking skills, excellent listening skills, attention to detail, mental alertness, and in-depth medical knowledge are all important traits for the HDS to possess. (Refer to Chapter 1: Professional Development.)

Obstacles including heavy foreign accents, poor speech habits, and speech defects, such as a lisp, complicate the process for both the HDS and the SR software. Although an HDS can **"flag"** a report as unintelligible, the SR software will translate the unintelligible word(s) from the existing database of **"learned" language**. The result is often either a **"word salad"** or missing text. These flaws trigger concerns that SRT could have adverse effects on patient care, creating the demand for highly qualified HDSs. The HDS simultaneously listens, reads, and edits to create an accurate and complete legal medical record. Every word must be confirmed in this process. Thus, the HDS is essential to healthcare documentation insofar as accuracy, consistency, and risk management are concerned.

See Appendix G for more resources related to medical and SR errors and case studies.

SPEECH WRECK FUNNIES

Speech recognition editing is serious business and shouldn't be taken lightly, but it is not uncommon to encounter some amusing mishaps put out by SR engines, often termed "speech wreck." It's not a crime to laugh and lighten the mood, just make sure you edit the text appropriately before moving on to the next report.

Here are some fun examples of speech wreck:

SR: The patient has 1-2 buttock martinis daily.

 D: The patient has 1-2 vodka martinis daily.

SR: The patient is a grocery store stalker.

 D: The patient is a grocery store stocker.

SR: She says she had an appendectomy and Candida.

 D: She says she had an appendectomy in Canada.

SR: The patient is scheduled for a Valium stress test.

 D: The patient is scheduled for a thallium stress test.

SR: His family is accepting of the fact that he has difficulties with academics, such as not passing enough gas and not doing well.

 D: His family is accepting of the fact that he has difficulties with academics, such as not passing FCATs and not doing well.

SR: Bowel sounds are pregnant x4 quadrants.

 D: Bowel sounds are present x4 quadrants.

SR: Case was discussed orally with her on the phone.

 D: Case was discussed thoroughly with her on the phone.

SR: Positive for increased throat.

 D: Positive for increased thirst.

MORE DICTATION MISADVENTURES

Not all speech recognition errors are funny. Sometimes what is dictated comes out sounding inappropriate or incorrect. Such words and phrases should be edited for clarity, sent to the QA department, or otherwise brought to the dictator's attention. (Also see Chapter 3: Using Good Judgment)

 D: Note, the patient has eloped from the hospital, and this psychiatric evaluation is being done in the patient's absence.

 D: Term gestation complicated by twin gestation and a premature birth.

 D: They do have a cat in the house, which she states is an outdoor animal.

 D: He states usually when he gets drunk, he feels like committing suicide but has never followed through.

 D: We could not get much history from the patient since he is comatose.

 D: Minimize blood loss to avoid blood loss.

 D: She does report being G1, P1, with a history of a term spontaneous vaginal delivery of a 2-year-old male.

 D: (Patient presented with vaginal bleeding) She has not had anything in her vagina in some time.

 D: On speculum exam: I completely cauterized. Did not see any other bleeding. Waited 5 minutes; still did not see any bleeding. She looks great.

 D: The patient consents to suture repair verbally.

 D: The walking is worse with activity.

 D: The patient is a 12-week-old pregnant patient who presents to the emergency department tonight with vomiting.

 D: Facial trauma is limited to the face.

 D: I told the mom to encourage fluids. I did encourage her to burp between each breast.

 D: The patient complained of headache this morning and then had sudden loss of consciousness, screaming out in pain.

 D: (Regarding a laceration to the lip) It is superficial but full-thickness.

 D: The patient is an otherwise healthy African American 13-year-old Caucasian male.

 D: She denies any unknown heavy lifting.

 D: The patient does not smoke alcohol or drink drugs.

 D: His right upper extremity is sent for x-ray of the elbow and forearm.

UNIT 3

ELEMENTS OF MEDICAL EDITING

CHAPTER 6

BUILDING EDITING SKILLS

KEY TERMS

assimilation
auditor
carpal tunnel syndrome
contextual content
dictator profiles
homonyms

macros
over-editing
proprietary platforms
repetitive-use injuries
track changes

LEARNING OBJECTIVES

1. Identify at least three benefits of using speech recognition.

2. Name the three skills used in the medical editor role and how they work together.

3. Restate what types of tools are used in medical editing and how they or their use may differ from traditional transcription.

4. Summarize the meaning of using active listening skills and provide several examples.

5. Analyze how accuracy and clarity should be maintained in edited speech-recognized documents.

6. Define "contextual content" and provide examples of the three different types noted.

7. Show three types of edits that *should* be made against three types of superfluous edits.

INTRODUCTION

Years ago stenographers took down dictation by hand to document reports. They were present in offices, operating rooms, and in morgues. The medical record has always been sacrosanct. Over time, technology has advanced and improved, giving us new tools that help from a technology standpoint. Speech recognition is one such tool that enriches the work environment.

Benefits of Speech Recognition

Some of the benefits to utilizing SR technology include a decreased risk of **carpal tunnel syndrome** and **repetitive-use injuries** resulting from physical strain. On the flip side, medical editing using SR technology can be both physically and mentally demanding. Some HDSs feel less physically tired at the end of their workday but more "brain dead." The reason for this is that medical editing often requires an HDS to be more engaged in the report than when performing traditional transcription.

Benefits to the medical editing process include the ability for increasing medical vocabularies when learning new accounts and specialties. Editing is most often faster than transcribing, and SR

SR BLOOPERS

While editing medical records is very serious business and is not to be taken lightly, draft text produced by SR engines can often add humor to an HDS's day. Bloopers such as:

SR: DISCHARGE INSTRUCTIONS: No lifting or bending, at least until this improves or until he is deceased.

D: DISCHARGE INSTRUCTIONS: No lifting or bending, at least until this improves or until he is <u>released</u>.

SR: (In a medication list) She attacked 10 mg.

D: <u>Zyrtec</u> 10 mg.

SR: The risks discussed included deep venous Moses.

D: The risks discussed included deep venous <u>thrombosis</u>.

SR: PAST MEDICAL HISTORY: Excision of left leg aliens.

D: PAST MEDICAL HISTORY: Excision of left <u>ganglion cyst</u>.

---

engines can "assist" when learning new accounts that have established dictators. For example, good **dictator profiles** that have been built up can be an effective way for the new HDS to become exposed to terminology that will enhance their knowledge and experience.

Changes in the Work Environment

In medical editing, the draft document produced by the SR engine is available immediately in its entirety. Therefore, editors can scan the document to look for obvious formatting errors—such as lists or paragraphs out of alignment or unused headers that should be removed. Since this can be a distraction, do a quick pre-edit. By pre-editing for obvious format changes prior to listening to the dictation, editors can stay with the flow of audio and concentrate on the words they are hearing and seeing on the screen instead of having to stop to make formatting changes.

Editors should approach their work with the very realistic expectation that something to edit will appear in every document. After all, this is your role as a medical editor: listening, reading, and editing. Listening skills become even more important when editing and require a different skill set from traditional transcription where the audio goes in the ears and out the fingers. With editing, audio goes from the ears to the eyes to the fingers. HDSs must make sure what their eyes are reading is what their ears are hearing; they need to make sure their fingers accurately reflect those edits to words on the screen. The process for listening, reading, and interpreting is more critical with editing than with straight transcription. This is why the medical editor must stay focused, not relying heavily on electronic devices.

THE MECHANICS

Cut the Proverbial Cord

In traditional transcription it is common to use keyboard shortcuts and a word expansion program to save keystrokes, which in turn saves time and boosts production. This is pretty easy to do when transcribing a medical record because you can quickly breeze through the demographics as well as the rest of the report—when the dictator does not jump around from section to section, that is. Your mouse is there when you need to maneuver to different screens or to pull up the Internet to verify a word. For the most part, your hands have no reason to leave the keyboard until you move on to the next report.

In medical editing, emphasis also is placed on the keyboard, but knowledge and skills of keyboard shortcuts must be taken to the next level. Some of those shortcuts may be utilized in traditional transcription, but in editing speech-recognized documents, your eyes are following along but your fingers are not—there is a lot more jumping around from one place to another. There is less typing of words or phrases and more utilization of the function and arrow keys, so navigating and editing by using keystrokes will help with efficiency and productivity.

So what time is it? It is time to get "mouse broken"; that is, to break the habit of reaching for the mouse when a keyboard shortcut can—make that *should*—be used. While there may be specific things within specific platforms that can be done only with a mouse, if there *is* a keystroke available to perform the same function, it will be faster than using the mouse. Here's why: By taking your hands off the keyboard, you are losing two to three seconds per edit. That may not sound like a lot, but multiply that by the number of edits made using the mouse per report, then take that times the number of reports you complete every day, every week, and every pay period. It quickly adds up.

Text Expanders

Text or word expansion programs have probably been the most important efficiency tool to healthcare documentation specialists, secondary only to our brains. These programs produce complete words, phrases, and paragraphs in an instant with minimal taps on the keyboard.

There are a number of text expander programs on the market, a list of which can be found in Appendix G: Resources. Many companies utilize Microsoft Word for transcription and editing, in which case AutoCorrect and AutoText options are built in and available for use—though most other text expansion programs will also work within the Microsoft Office Suite products as well as some other **proprietary platforms**. If you have purchased and use a particular word expansion program, be sure to check with potential employers to find out if it will be compatible with the platform on which you will be working.

Word expansion programs can still be useful in editing medical reports, even though you may not use all of your 4,000 (or more) entries as with straight transcription. Word expansion programs are generally versatile, so you most likely will be able to create shortcuts equally as impressive in almost any program. Check the Help section, User's Guide, or manufacturer's website for help in creating specific shortcuts.

ENSURING ACCURACY

As mentioned in the Knowledge Is Power section of Chapter 1, listening and *editing* a medical report is a different skill set than listening and *transcribing*. Words seen on the screen have the power to influence more so than typing them from scratch. Resist the temptation to go on autopilot. As in traditional transcription, accuracy of edited documents must be maintained.

In editing, the HDS must *think* quickly more so than type quickly, so knowledge of medical terminology is even more critical during the editing process. The HDS must be able to listen and move through the document efficiently and recognize when a word or medication is out of context.

Use Active Listening Skills

Using active listening skills means listening for contextual meaning or content. Absorb the meaning of what is being dictated—listen for what is meant, not just what is said. This will help to identify and avoid errors being recorded. Here are some tips to effectively use active listening skills:

- **Minimize external distractions.** Work in a quiet environment in which you can hear the dictation well and not be distracted by the TV, phone calls, children playing, and so on.
- **Focus solely on what the dictator is saying.** Concentrate on listening and matching the words being spoken with what you are reading on the screen.
- **Minimize internal distractions.** Clear your mind of everything except the task at hand. You cannot give your full attention to your work if you are thinking about errands you need to run or daydreaming about an upcoming vacation. Quickly jotting down to-dos on a piece of paper will free up your thoughts to return to work worry-free. This will help you feel organized and focused on the work at hand.
- **Keep an open mind.** Evaluate statements made for accuracy and consistency but wait until the end of the dictation to draw conclusions. Illuminating details are often revealed as you get further through the report.
- **Engage yourself.** Keep a notebook and pen handy to jot down questions or potential inconsistencies that need to be checked. This is being thorough.

The Power of Suggestion

The power of suggestion is assuming what is heard and seen on the screen is the same; in reality, it may or may not be so. It is easy to assume what is seen on our screen is what is heard. It is important to make sure to read each and every word individually as you are editing. Sound-alike words, assimilated words, and accents all have the power to alter what is understood by the HDS.

There are medical and nonmedical sound-alike words and **homonyms** frequently used in medicine. Make sure the words seen on the screen are correct based on the **contextual content**. Examples include:

- ACE versus ace versus Ace
- acidic versus ascetic versus acetic
- affect versus effect
- breech versus breach

- enuresis versus anuresis
- heal versus heel
- liver versus livor
- know versus no
- oral versus aural
- track versus tract

Also see Appendix B: Challenging Words, Terms, and Prefixes.

Assimilation is the influence of a sound on a neighboring sound so that the two become similar or the same. However, a huge difference lies in the meanings of assimilated words, so pay close attention to other clues in the report. Examples include:

- competent versus incompetent
- febrile versus afebrile
- possible versus impossible
- aspirated versus separated
- oozing versus using
- procedure informed versus procedure performed

As outlined in Chapter 3: Deciphering Accents, unfamiliar speech, tones, and syllables all play a role in the SR engine's ability to accurately capture what is spoken and in the HDS's ability to edit text. Other nuances of accents factor in as well. Examples include:

- Unusual pronunciation and phrasing
- Incorrect usage of words and phrases
- Repetitious speech
- Hesitations and pauses
- Speed of voice on dictation

Complete "The Power of Intervention" exercise in the box below to test yourself.

Over-Editing

Use the draft speech-recognized document to first make quick editing decisions, resolve blanks, predict edits, and remove unnecessary content that should not be included (e.g., sidebar conversations recorded by SR engine that are accidentally added to the report).

Corrections made to a draft that make it more readable but have no effect on the medical accuracy or meaning is considered **over-editing**. Over-editing can actually send bad information back to the SR engine when it goes through adaptation (the SR engine's process of "learning"). Do not get caught up in over-editing grammar, punctuation, style, and readability. As long as the critical details are clear and accurately captured or edited, complete sentences and incorrect grammar or punctuation that has *no* impact on medical meaning or clarity of the record may fall by the wayside. This can be a difficult concept for the experienced HDS to accept and why some struggle to transition from traditional transcription to editing efficiently and seamlessly. It can cause some to fail to meet editing quotas. Over-editing can affect the HDS's paycheck.

For example: In transcription school or in learning on the job, many students were instructed to include "The" before "patient" even if "patient" was all that was dictated. In medical editing, avoid making such changes that are solely style-based and have no negative medical impact on the integrity of the document. Adding the word "the" is considered over-editing because it gives no extra value to the statement; it simply makes it smoother to read.

In the Example of Over-editing box on page 42, unnecessary extra words were added by the HDS. The HDS did not need to expand "2L O_2" and could have simply inserted semicolons to separate phrases. Alternately, the phrases could have been separated into sentences. For example: Patient monitored. Given 2L O_2, Tylenol, albuterol. Admitted. Moved to floor.

Examine how an edit can be made with the fewest number of keystrokes while maintaining the medical integrity and intended meaning of the document. Again, do not add words simply to

---

EXERCISE: THE POWER OF INTERVENTION

Read the following examples and determine the correct term by avoiding the power of suggestion and instead using critical thinking skills.

1. He should have colonoscopy within 2 beers.

2. The patient is 63 unhappy inches tall.

3. She was in the Army and was in training to become a manic.

4. The patient had suicidal polyps.

5. There was a 2 cm lesion on the left labia menorah.

> ### EXAMPLE OF OVER-EDITING
>
> **D:** Patient monitored, given 2L O$_2$, Tylenol, albuterol, admitted, moved to floor.
>
> **T:** The patient was monitored; given 2 liters of oxygen, Tylenol, and albuterol; admitted and moved to the floor.

make the text more readable. The HDS is helping to create a legal medical record, not an essay or a short story.

When to Edit

Always edit when there is a doubt, such as:

- Left/right discrepancies
- Pronoun discrepancies (he/she)
- Inconsistent lab results
- Inconsistent medication dosages

Always leave a blank and/or flag the report if you cannot verify and rectify the discrepancy (follow facility or client policies and procedures).

It can be more efficient to slow down; it is not always more productive to speed up. Slowing down allows time to make edits and to keep up with the dictation. By using navigational and editing keystrokes, you will avoid taking your fingers off the keyboard to use the mouse. Thus, the tools used will produce the speed.

Learning to edit is like learning any new skill. When you first started transcribing, you had to practice a lot. It can also take time to learn to edit efficiently. Start with a few navigational and editing keyboard shortcuts, and then add shortcuts when the previous ones have been mastered. Every platform has numerous keystrokes, though the types of keystrokes programmed or allowed may differ. The HDS should pick the ones likely to be used most often and learn those first to increase skill level. This process is similar to assigning and learning **macros** within a word-expansion program.

A lot of platforms, especially Microsoft Word-based platforms, use keystrokes that are the same as in Word. Some of these keystrokes will transfer over for use in email, browsers, and other documents being used. By increasing your knowledge of keyboard shortcuts, you will reap the benefits not only in the work environment but also in your personal environment. Editing can be much more than learning a new process; it can lead to an easier way of working overall.

Proofreading Tips

As a healthcare documentation specialist (HDS), proofreading is one of the most important aspects of the job—whether doing traditional transcription or speech-recognized medical editing.

An interesting facet of proofreading is getting the human brain to see what is actually on the page while simultaneously reading content and listening to the playback of the recorded voice file. Our brains tend to see what we know should be there instead of what actually appears on the screen—especially if we are experienced and have transcribed hundreds of vaginal deliveries, appendectomies, or radiology reports, for example. The challenge is to read one word at a time and for our brains to see one word at a time; in this way, every detail is observed. Sometimes it helps to start proofreading in reverse—from the last word on the page to the first. This keeps our brains from getting lost in the content.

Keep the following tips in mind when proofing and editing medical reports:

- Proofreading includes medical terms, English words, upper case or lower case, punctuation, spacing, style, and formatting.
- The HDS or medical editor is expected to keep the grammar, punctuation, and sentence structure correct regardless of what is dictated; however, the medical meaning of any part of a report cannot be changed.
- For errors that affect the medical meaning, flag the report for review by QA, an **auditor**, or the dictating physician. An underscored blank should be left for dictation that has been garbled or is unclear for any reason. Dictated reports are sometimes labeled "dictated but not read" or "signed but not read." Therefore, we know the HDS or medical editor is being depended upon for accuracy.
- Remember: What is *not* an error is just as important to know as what *is* an error. These details can change depending upon circumstances, the reference material utilized, and the wishes of the employer or client. The HDS or medical editor should stay up-to-date with changes in the profession. Be flexible.
- When transitioning from student to employee or from one job to another, keep and use all handouts provided on the job that refer to transcription, style, formatting, editing, and so on, in order to properly transcribe or edit and proofread reports for your employer or client.

- Each employer or client may have different requirements for the HDS independent contractor. Create a folder with all pertinent documents for each one in either hard copy or electronic copy formats. A hard copy is easy to add notes to quickly and can easily be referenced, while an electronic copy could be quickly searched using CTRL + F. While some may prefer to keep both hard and electronic copies, this can double the work by having to make each update in two places. Whichever your preference, be sure to review these documents on a regular basis for necessary changes, and do not forget to back up your files.

N.B.: Some proofreading can involve **track changes**. Tutorials regarding track changes can be found on YouTube and the Microsoft website.

Style and Formatting Tips

Keep the following style and formatting tips in mind when editing medical reports:

- *Patient names*: Preference is to use "patient" or "the patient" instead of typing the name as dictated—unless your employer/client insists the patient name be used when dictated.
- *Numbers*: Preference is to use arabic numerals as much as possible, especially for technical information such as measurements, dosages, and so on. Be mindful, however, of two numbers next to each other (Example: two 5 mL syringes; 10 one-inch items).
- *Dates*: Spell out the date at the top of a letter. The number format with a four-digit year may be used in a medical report. There are several correct date styles; stay consistent throughout each report with your date style, whether spelling it out or using the number format—traditional or military style.

- *Spacing*: Using one space after a sentence is preferred, but using two is not wrong. While it is always better to be consistent, it is unnecessary to adjust dictation templates to match specific styles or vice versa. Use one space after the period at the end of an abbreviation, after a colon used as punctuation in a sentence, and after the D and T lines in a sign-off block.
- *Special Characters*: This depends on what software program is being used. Some will accept characters like %, #, < >, and °, but others will not; in which case these must be spelled out when dictated: percent, number, greater than/less than, degree, and so on.

QUALITY ASSURANCE

Quality assurance (QA) provides a bridge between healthcare documentation specialists, supervisors, and dictating physicians. QA specialists, sometimes called auditors, proofread the completed work, correct it when necessary, and give feedback to each HDS. In this way, individual employees are helped in their learning process of specialized medical terminology and the individual dictators' styles. Management, in turn, is helped in their evaluation process. The organization overall and patients alike are helped by each HDS then applying what he or she learned from QA feedback to future reports, which increases the overall quality and efficiency. QA feedback and reminders are best accomplished through individual audits as well as through monthly meetings or newsletters. Every organization should have a QA department that performs at least quarterly audits of all transcription/editing staff.

UNIT 4

REPORT TYPES

CHAPTER 7

CORRESPONDENCE

KEY TERMS

block format
modified block format
semi-block format

LEARNING OBJECTIVES

1. List notable differences between a correspondence letter and other report types.

2. Name the three format styles for letters and identify the major style differences.

3. Identify elements of a correspondence letter also included in other report types.

4. Discuss the differences between letters and memoranda and the purposes for which each is best suited.

INTRODUCTION

Whereas HDSs most often edit report types in the "basic four,"—which includes history and physical examinations, consultations, operative reports, and discharge summaries—the occasional letter or memorandum will present itself in the queue for editing. Physicians and their assistants dictate letters and memoranda for a variety of reasons. The types of correspondence included in this chapter will give the medical editing student a balanced exposure to and understanding of this aspect of the career field. See the following model reports for examples of a memorandum and a followup letter. See "Formatting Letters" on page 47 for more details.

CRITICAL THINKING EXERCISE 7-1

Physicians dictate medications to be given via specific routes. Intradermal, subcutaneous, percutaneous, and per os are examples of routes of administration. What effect might it have if an incorrect route of administration were transcribed in a medical report?

MODEL REPORTS

~ INTEROFFICE M E M O ~

To: QualiCare Clinic Staff

From: Human Resources

Re: Preparing for Joint Commission on 28 April ----

Date: 19 March ----

Two of the steps that must be taken in preparation for Joint Commission include:

(1) Each member of the QualiCare Clinic staff is required to read and sign the current edition of our Policy & Procedure Handbook.

(2) Each member of the staff must have an up-to-date tuberculosis test with results posted no later than 19 April.

Please keep in mind that the deadline for each of the above is **19 April**, regardless of shift or schedule. If any member of the staff feels this deadline cannot be met, please see your supervisor immediately.

Thank you for your cooperation. Working together, I feel sure we will have an excellent result from our Joint Commission audit.

10 March ----

Michael Panagides, MD, Internal Medicine
5630 Tulip Poplar Lane
Nashville, TN 37212

Patient Name: Marlena Reed
DOB: 01/14/----
Patient ID: REE027

Dear Dr. Panagides:

The patient is a 66-year-old Caucasian woman accompanied today by her husband. Medical problems include multinodular/cystic thyroid, osteoporosis, and estrogen replacement therapy. She returns for management of thyroid, endocrine, and medical problems.

She saw Dr. Tomas 02/29/---- for "dizzy," had 2-D echocardiogram 03/01/----, and is wearing an event monitor for 30 days. She will see Dr. Tomas again 03/31/----.

The patient states she has "dizzy vertigo when I get up and turn fast." She saw Dr. Roberts last week for her glaucoma check, which she has done every 4 months. She will see Dr. Roberts again in July.

She saw Dr. Ellis on 01/25/---- and reported that he wanted her to stay on Premarin. She will see Dr. Ellis again in 6 months.

I reviewed the laboratory data from 01/15/---- with the patient and her husband. All questions were answered to their satisfaction.

DXA bone density study on 02/26/---- showed osteoporosis. There is a suggestion of anterior wedging at vertebrae T9 and T10. The LVA analysis was impaired by her scoliosis and marked osteoporosis at her lumbar vertebral bodies. Therefore, the computer label of "compression fracture at L2 and L3" is not reliable. Her overall 10-year fracture risk was 29% and hip fracture risk 7%. DXA data from 02/26/---- is compared to that of 08/20/----. Statistically, no significant changes are in evidence.

(Continued)

Michael Panagides, MD, Internal Medicine
Patient Name: Marlena Reed
Date of Consult: 10 Mar ----
Page 2

Thyroid sonogram also done on 02/26/---- showed a 0.5 × 0.2 × 0.3 cm nodule in the right lobe and a 0.3 × 0.2 × 0.21 cm nodule in the left lobe.

At this time I will recommend recheck of a thyroid sonogram in 6 months. For her osteoporosis, I will recommend continued Fosamax treatment until 05/01/---- before considering the possibility of a "drug holiday." We will maintain her vitamin D at optimal levels. She will continue calcium supplements. We discussed a trial off Premarin, and she agreed to discuss this with Dr. Ellis at her next appointment. I also would like Ms. Reed to enroll in an exercise class, specifically for tai chi, which is a regimen that helps with balance. She agreed to consider this.

Thank you for the opportunity to assist in the care of this pleasant lady. Please let me know if I can offer further diagnostic or therapeutic recommendations.

Best regards,

Yancy Rhodes, MD, Endocrinology

YR:xx
D: 3/10/----
T: 3/10/----

C: Esteban Tomas, MD, Cardiology
   Ronald L. Roberts, MD, Ophthalmology
   Marcus Ellis, MD, Obstetrics/Gynecology

STYLES AND STANDARDS

When clinicians need to dictate correspondence it is usually in the form of a letter to consulting or referring physicians, insurance companies, attorneys, or employees. In traditional transcription, unless a facility or client preferred that the correspondence be entirely in narrative paragraph style, it most often would follow the same format as a consultation report.

A physician may need to dictate only an update about a patient involved in a car accident who has finished physical therapy or dictate a school excuse for no physical education for a patient with a broken leg. Letters may be longer, containing more detailed information for complex cases, such as a patient with a prolonged respiratory illness who has undergone extensive laboratory and diagnostic testing and taken multiple courses of antibiotics, steroids, and breathing treatments. Letters may be dictated to consultants who are friends; therefore, first names may be used in the salutation and in the closing.

No matter the length or reason for the correspondence, the HDS should take care to edit with as much focus and attention to detail as any other report type.

Consultation reports typically include findings of the consultant's independent physical examination of the patient as well as diagnostic studies, laboratories, and treatments. The consultant's assessment or diagnosis of the patient will be given along with their recommendations or plan for the patient moving forward.

Formatting Letters

Consultation reports, and thus correspondence letters (printed on office stationery), typically include the sender's address, date, recipient's address, salutation, body, closing, signature, enclosures, transcriptionist's initials, and carbon copy notation (if any).

Patient demographic information, along with the sender's and recipient's addresses, may or may not be imported into the letter, depending on the type of platform being used and whether correspondence letters are part of the platform's implementation package.

Speech-recognized letters are formatted according to a template; however, if no template is available, they may need to be edited. A correspondence letter is most often brief and only one page long. However, this will depend on to whom the letter is being sent as well as the amount and nature of information required. Remember, if a second page

is necessary, "(Continued)" must be entered at the end of page one. Page two must contain at least two lines of text from the body of the letter. Do not leave a signature line alone on page two.

Keep in mind that correspondence letters being viewed in an electronic environment may not require subsequent page headers; scrolling down the page may be all that is needed. However, when letters are written in a program such as Microsoft Word with the intention of being emailed or printed, formatting for continuation pages as noted above should be followed.

Three types of formats are typically used in correspondence: block, modified block, and semi-block. Again, which type will depend on the platform being used and facility or client preference.

Block format is the most common type of business letter layout. The entire letter is justified left and single-spaced except for double spacing between paragraphs.

Modified block format is another popular layout. In this type, the sender's and recipient's addresses as well as the body of the letter are justified left, but the date and closing are tabbed to the center of the page.

Semi-block format is the least common style of layout used. It is similar to the modified block format except that each paragraph is indented instead of flush left.

It will not be necessary to change the font size or type, as these are typically programmed into the platform and customized according to the client's preference.

In a business setting, insert a colon (:) after the salutation, and insert a comma (,) after the closing. If the originator dictates the salutation by first name, use a comma instead of a colon after the salutation. Be sure to include the HDS's initials at the bottom of the report and include any copy or enclosure information provided. Many times the date and time stamps for auditing purposes are automatically populated by the electronic medical record system.

Examples of salutations and closings used in letters are listed in Table 7-1.

CRITICAL THINKING EXERCISE 7-2

While teaching a class, you are asked if there are any prerequisites or conditions necessary before a patient can undergo gastric bypass surgery. How would you respond?

TABLE 7-1 EXAMPLES OF SALUTATIONS AND CLOSINGS USED IN LETTERS

Dear Dr. Thomas:	Dear Bill,
Most sincerely,	Best wishes,
David Smith, MD, General Surgery	("Dave" is dictated and will be handwritten.)
	David Smith, MD, General Surgery (transcribed)
DS:xx	DS:xx
C: Jane Doe, MD, Infectious Disease	C: Jane Doe, MD, Infectious Disease
Encl: Lab results	Encl: Lab results

Formatting Memoranda

Like letters, memoranda are used for a variety of reasons, including notices to employees, information to be distributed to a board of directors, or a change or update in policies and procedures for an office or institution. In some cases, a memo sent to office personnel will have to be verified as having been received by each employee. Keep a folder of memos for future reference, especially for training new employees.

Memos are formatted very simply. Using company stationery, center the word MEMORAN-DUM in all caps at least two to four blank lines down from the logo. Enter "To," "From," "RE" or "Re" (for *regarding*), and "Date" double-spaced and flush with the left margin, adding the appropriate information following each heading. Tab from the colons following each heading for a neat, easily readable line of information. Space down another two to four blank lines and begin the memo proper. Adjust the spacing to keep the information vertically centered on the page. Double-space paragraphs. No signature line is necessary because the originator initials the "From" line. In some instances, the HDS might enter the initials at the bottom of the page to identify the originator and transcriptionist. This would depend upon the nature of the memo and its distribution list.

INDEX OF CORRESPONDENCE REPORTS

Student Name: _____   Date: _____

ID Number	Name	Type of Report/Procedure
C-1	Rebecca Barton	Cover letter
C-2	Rebecca Barton	Thank-you letter
C-3	Elizabeth Stapley	Letter of reference
C-4	Donna Hayes	Letter of reference
C-6	Arlene Scarborough	Letter to SAT Program Coordinator
C-7	Ronald Williams	Followup letter, surgical patient
C-8	Sierra Collins	Followup letter, surgical patient
C-9	Jessie Garza	Followup letter, surgical patient
C-10	William R. Barker	Followup letter, surgical patient
C-11	Melinda E. Parker	Followup letter, surgical patient
C-12	Tyler C. Thompson	Followup letter, surgical patient
C-13	Corina Gomez	Followup letter, surgical patient
C-14	Rob Skinner	Followup letter, surgical patient
C-15	Curtis Gravell	Followup letter, surgical patient
C-16	Gene Falcon	Followup letter, Hematology/Oncology
C-17	Hilda Cordova	Followup letter, Hematology/Oncology
C-18	Scott Cash	Followup letter, Hematology/Oncology
C-19	Jaime Villarreal	Followup letter, Hematology/Oncology
C-20	Marie Luz Cortez	Followup letter, Hematology/Oncology
C-21	Nancy Froment	Followup letter, Hematology/Oncology
C-22	Cody Scott	Followup letter, Hematology/Oncology
C-23	Rhonda Brown	Followup letter, Hematology/Oncology
C-24	Thomas Wayne Crawford	Letter to lawyer
C-25	Wendy Davis	Followup letter, dermatology patient
C-26	Carrie Lynn Rogers	Followup letter, surgical patient
C-28	Denise Renee Carver	Followup letter, endocrinology patient
C-29	Tracy Leigh Schneider	Followup letter, cardiology patient
C-30	Michael Weston	Followup letter, cardiology patient
C-31	Mary Graham-Morris	Interoffice memo
C-32	Karl S. Woods	Memorandum

CHAPTER 8

RADIOLOGY

LEARNING OBJECTIVES

1. Define telemedicine and give three benefits this service offers the field of radiology.
2. Learn the differences between BI-RADS, HI-RADS, and LI-RADS.
3. Explain how density of the breast can affect a mammogram result.
4. Describe how electrodes are numbered in electroencephalogram reports.
5. Learn formatting necessary in electrocardiogram reports.
6. Learn the different specialties that employ ultrasonography in diagnostic radiology.

INTRODUCTION

Radiology is that branch of the health sciences that deals with radioactive substances and radiant energy, together with the diagnosis and treatment of disease by means of roentgen rays (x-rays) or ultrasound techniques. The radiology report is a description of the findings and the interpretation of radiographs and other studies done by a radiologist. A radiologist is a physician who has been certified in Diagnostic Radiology by The American Board of Radiology.

In this text we have included interventional radiology and nuclear medicine as well as mammography, ultrasonography, computed tomography (CT), magnetic resonance angiography (MRA), magnetic resonance imaging (MRI), and sonography to give the medical editing student a broad introduction to this vital field of medicine. It is not intended to be an all-inclusive list, as the field of radiology is growing and expanding constantly through research.

Radiology is an integral area of medicine that assists in confirming or refuting a suspected diagnosis of a patient. Large healthcare facilities such as hospitals have in-house radiology services, while smaller clinics and physician offices generally write orders for their patients to have diagnostic studies performed at an independent radiology center. Depending on the specialty, certain diagnostic studies may be performed in the office. For example, cardiologists can perform an electrocardiogram (EKG or ECG) or an echocardiogram in their office to help determine heart function and whether or not disease is present. Likewise, an obstetrician can perform an in-office ultrasound to visualize the embryo or fetus to obtain a variety of health information about the baby and the mother, such as gestational age, rotation of the uterus, or placenta previa. *N.B.:* All reports in this text can be dictated in both inpatient and outpatient settings.

Telemedicine is an increasingly popular service used by clinicians for remote radiologic services or remote patient monitoring, especially during nighttime hours when personnel staffing is minimal or in rural areas where full-time radiologists are cost-prohibitive. Teleradiology technologies make it possible for studies such as x-rays, CT scans, and MRIs to be read in a timely and secure manner.

In addition, front-end speech recognition (FESR) is widely used in radiology. Language used in diagnostic studies is highly repetitive, making FESR ideal for use with this specialty. A quality review process is an important step in maintaining accuracy, and it should still be in place and performed upon clinician-created documentation by either the dictator or an HDS.

See the following model reports for examples of different radiology reports. See Formatting Radiology Reports on page 54 for more details.

A&P BRAIN DRAIN BOX 8-1

What are the three functions of the vertebral column?

MODEL REPORT 1: RADIOLOGY

CT SCAN OF CHEST WITHOUT CONTRAST

Patient Name: Peggy Campbell   **Referring Physician**: Tonya Warren, MD
DOB: 11/09/----   **Date of Exam**: 06/04/----
Sex/Age: F/70   **Patient ID**: R-3401

HISTORY: Patient presents with a cough. She has had previous surgery for left-sided breast cancer.

FINDINGS: Areas of pleural calcification and pleural thickening are seen in the left hemithorax, the distribution being consistent with prior asbestos exposure. Focal chronic fibrosis is seen in the left lower lobe with generalized hyperinflation of the lungs suggesting chronic obstructive pulmonary disease.

A 5.7 mm, somewhat lobulated mass is seen in the right middle lobe that could be a noncalcified granuloma or could represent a very small primary lung tumor or a solitary metastatic lesion. I would recommend a followup CT scan in 6 months for further evaluation.

The heart size is minimally enlarged. No focal infiltrates seen in the lungs. No hilar or mediastinal adenopathy.

The liver, spleen, pancreas, adrenal glands, upper poles of both kidneys, and biliary ducts are WNL. The gallbladder is not imaged.

IMPRESSION
1. Areas of pleural thickening and pleural calcification are seen in the left hemithorax, suggesting prior asbestos exposure.
2. A 5.7 mm, somewhat lobulated mass is noted in the right middle lobe. This could represent a malignant or benign process. Patient has had previous surgery for left-sided breast cancer.
3. Hyperinflation of the lungs, indicating chronic obstructive pulmonary disease, is also seen, along with chronic fibrosis in the left lung base.
4. The heart size is minimally enlarged.

RECOMMENDATIONS: I would recommend a followup CT scan in 6 months to ensure stability.

Thank you for this outpatient referral.

Electronically signed by Grayson Bruckman, MD, Radiology, on 06/04/---- at 1800 hours.

GB:xx
DD: 06/04/----
DT: 06/04/----

C: Tonya Warren, MD, Hematology/Oncology
   Robert Altman, MD, Pulmonary Surgery/Respiratory Medicine

MODEL REPORT 2

MRI, LUMBAR SPINE

Patient Name: Tracy D. Ashbaugh   **Referring Physician**: Holly Russo, MD
DOB: 05/10/----   **Date of Study**: 12/15/----
Sex/Age: F/40   **Patient ID**: R-9355

HISTORY: Low back pain in a 40-year-old white female.

TECHNIQUE: Multiplanar imaging (sagittal, axial, and/or coronal planes) was performed using various scanning parameters (T1- and T2-wSE, +/-FS, GE, and/or IR techniques).

FINDINGS: A normal lumbar lordosis is seen. No intramedullary bony lesions are present. No evidence of intrathecal lesions, intraspinal or paraspinal masses, and no spinal stenosis. The conus is at the T12-L1 level. No fracture is seen.

At the L1-2 level, the disk space is maintained. The disk is well hydrated with no evidence of herniation.

At the L2-3 level, the disk space is maintained. The disk is well hydrated with no evidence of herniation.

At the L3-4 level, the disk space is maintained. The disk is well hydrated with no evidence of herniation. Neural foramina are patent. No degenerative spurring of facet joints noted.

At the L4-5 level, the disk space is maintained. The disk is well hydrated with no evidence of herniation. Neural foramina are patent. No degenerative spurring of facet joints noted.

At the L5-S1 level, the disk space is maintained. Disk dehydration is noted. Posterior disk herniation with focal annular tear is impinging on the anterior thecal sac.

IMPRESSION: Disk herniation with annular tear, L5-S1.

Thank you for your kind referral.

_____
Charles Tew, MD, Diagnostic Radiology

CT:xx
DD: 12/15/----
DT: 12/16/----

C: Holly Russo, MD, Neurosurgery

MODEL REPORT 3

ROUTINE BILATERAL SCREENING MAMMOGRAMS

Patient Name: Jane Montgomery   **Referring Physician**: Murray Travis, MD
DOB: 10/22/----   **Date of Service**: 10/29/----
Age/Sex: 57/F   **Patient ID**: R-978

HISTORY: A 57-year-old black female with no palpable mass, no positive family history of breast cancer.

Digital mammographic views of the breasts were obtained and are compared to previous study of October last year. R2 CAD was used in review of this case.

The breasts show some scattered fibroglandular densities bilaterally. I see no spiculated dominant mass. No suspicious microcalcification, clustering, or skin thickening is noted. I see no significant change from the earlier study.

IMPRESSION
1. No dominant mass, suspicious calcification, or significant change from the prior study is seen. Annual mammographic followup is recommended.
2. BI-RADS Category 2: Benign finding.

This patient's calculated lifetime risk of breast cancer using the American Cancer Society's Gail assessment model is 6.4%. Recent American Cancer Society guidelines recommend screening breast MRI for patients with a risk assessment of 20% or greater.

This patient's BRCA analysis score was 0.1%. This is the calculated risk for this patient carrying the BRCA1 or BRCA2 genetic mutations. Our center recommends consideration of genetic counseling in patients with a 10% or higher score. The Diagnostic Imaging Center does offer genetic counseling services.

This study was reviewed with R2 CAD system.

NOTE: Mammography is only one portion of a complete breast evaluation, which also includes clinical breast exam and breast self-examination. Breast cancer may be obscured by overlying glandular tissue, especially in women with dense breasts.

(Continued)

Patient Name: Jane Montgomery
Date of Service: 10/29/----
Patient ID: R-978
Page 2

Ultrasound improves detection rates, but some cancers will not be detected even with the combination of mammography and ultrasound. Negative breast imaging should not preclude surgical biopsy of a clinically suspicious palpable finding.

Electronically signed by Grayson Bruckman, MD, Radiology, on 10/29/---- at 0915 hours.

GB:xx
D: 10/29/----
T: 10/29/----

C: Murray Travis, MD, Obstetrics/Gynecology

**This document has been dictated but not read and is subject to transcription variation.

MODEL REPORT 4

ULTRASOUND, PELVIS, COMPLETE/TRANSVAGINAL

Patient Name: Crystal T. Sommers   **Referring Physician**: C. W. Scott, MD
DOB: 10/28/----   **Date of Exam**: 03/20/----
Sex/Age: F/64   **Patient ID**: R-8801

HISTORY: Fibroid uterus.

COMPARISON STUDY: Pelvic sonogram done in February of last year.

TECHNIQUE: Transverse abdominal and transvaginal images.

FINDINGS: The uterus is enlarged, measuring 10.0 × 4.4 × 7.0 cm with its echotexture being heterogeneous. The endometrium, which is poorly visualized, measures 3 mm. In the lateral aspect of the uterine body, a 4.5 × 3.6 × 4.1 cm solid mass is seen, which is slightly larger compared to last year's study. In the midline, a 2.0 × 1.4 × 1.7 cm solid mass is unchanged. More inferiorly, a 2.0 × 1.1 × 1.9 solid mass has not changed since last year. On the left side of the uterine body is a 2.5 × 1.8 × 1.9 cm solid mass that has increased slightly since last year. Positioned within the fundus is a 1.9 × 1.0 × 1.9 cm solid mass indicative of a fibroid tumor that has not changed significantly. The right ovary measures 1.9 × 0.9 × 1.3 cm. The left ovary measures 1.8 × 1.4 × 1.5 cm and is unremarkable. Pulse Doppler interrogation of the ovaries demonstrates equal vascular flow.

IMPRESSION: Slightly enlarging fibroid tumors in an enlarged uterus, as described above.

Electronically signed by Grayson Bruckman, MD, Radiology, on 03/21/---- at 0855 hours.

GB:xx
DD: 03/20/----
DT: 03/20/----

C: Charles W. Scott, MD, OB/GYN

MODEL REPORT 5

NUCLEAR MEDICINE WHOLE-BODY THYROID SCAN

Patient Name: Constance Benavida   **Referring Physician**: Yancy Rhodes, MD
DOB: 06/04/----   **Date of Exam**: 09/11/----
Sex/Age: F/53   **Patient ID**: R-3114

HISTORY: 53-year-old Italian female with thyroid cancer, S/P thyroidectomy
6 weeks ago.

COMPARISON STUDY: None available.

TECHNIQUE: Patient was given 1.0 mCi of I-131 iodide orally, after which 48-hour
delayed whole-body images were obtained. Spot images were obtained over the
thyroid bed.

FINDINGS: A moderate amount of activity is seen in the thyroid bed indicating
residual thyroid tissue. This is felt to be WNL for this surgery. No extrathyroidal activity
is seen in the neck to indicate metastatic disease. Images of the whole-body show
a small amount of activity in the urinary bladder. This is felt to be physiologic. No
abnormal activity is seen.

IMPRESSION
1. Activity in the thyroid bed consistent with residual thyroid tissue.
2. No evidence of metastatic disease.

Thank you for this outpatient referral.

Electronically signed by Charles Tew, MD, Nuclear Medicine, on 9/11/---- at
1145 hours.

CT:xx
DD: 09/11/----
DT: 09/11/----

C: Yancy Rhodes, MD, Endocrinology

A&P BRAIN DRAIN BOX 8-2

List the three types of muscle tissue.

STYLES AND STANDARDS

As mentioned in Chapter 6: Building Editing Skills, while certain styles and standards such as grammar and punctuation are more relaxed in medical editing, the HDS should take care to maintain the integrity of the report, retain intended meaning, and format styles and standards related to radiology whenever possible. Students should refer to *The Book of Style for Medical Transcription*, other reputable resources, and facility or client preferences and guidelines related to styles and standards of radiology. Additional resources are also listed in Appendix G of this text.

Formatting Radiology Reports

While the general layout of radiology reports may vary based on facility or client preference, most reports include demographics information at the top and headings in all capitals followed by a colon and the body of the text on the same line. An alternate report format includes the headings in all capitals, with the body of the text beginning flush left on the line below the heading. No colon is included after the heading with this style.

Paragraphs are single-spaced and flush left, with double-spacing between paragraphs. Unused headings should be deleted. Numbered items of a list should each be placed on a separate line. The name or type of study is usually listed at the top of the report. Formatting of these reports can change depending upon employer and client wishes and/or platform requirements, so the HDS is advised to stay flexible on this issue.

Keep in mind that radiology reports being formatted and viewed in an electronic environment do not require page breaks or subsequent page headers because formatting is automatically generated by the technology. Follow facility guidelines to allow text to wrap from the beginning of the report to the end without adding page breaks.

Radiology reports that are formatted outside of an electronic environment or that will be printed should contain continuation information. For each subsequent page, "(Continued)" must be entered at the end of the page. The header at the top of the following page should contain the patient's name, medical record number (where applicable), the date of service, and the page number. Additional identifying information may be included in the header according to facility preference. Subsequent pages must contain at least two lines of text from the body of the report. Do not leave a signature line or a sign-off block alone on a page.

Model Report 3 in this chapter illustrates a report with continuation information. All other reports within this chapter are shown without page breaks or continuation information.

CRITICAL THINKING EXERCISE 8-1

While editing a preoperative History and Physical, the dictation shows that this type 1 diabetic pediatric patient is to be given 5 units/kg/day Humulin R prior to hammertoe surgery. This seems strange to you, and after checking your drug reference book, it is clear that this dose of Humulin R is incorrect. This is of concern. What should be done?

BI-RADS Categories

Mammogram reports

The American College of Radiology has developed a standard way of describing mammogram findings. In this system, the results are sorted into categories numbered 0 through 6. This system is called the *Breast Imaging Reporting and Data System* (BI-RADS), which is trademarked. Having a standard way of reporting mammogram results lets doctors use the same words and terms and ensures better followup of suspicious findings.

X-ray assessment is incomplete.
Category 0: Additional imaging evaluation and/or comparison to prior mammograms is needed.
This means a possible abnormality may not be clearly seen or defined and more tests are needed, such as the use of spot compression (applying compression to a smaller area when doing the mammogram), magnified views, special mammogram views, or ultrasound. This also suggests that the mammogram should be compared with older ones to see if there have been changes in the area over time.

X-ray assessment is complete.
Category 1: Negative.
There is no significant abnormality to report. The breasts look the same (they are symmetrical) with no masses (lumps), distorted structures, or suspicious calcifications. In this case, *negative* means nothing bad was found.

Category 2: Benign (non-cancerous) finding.
This is also a negative mammogram result (there is no sign of cancer), but the reporting doctor chooses to describe a finding known to be benign, such as benign calcifications, lymph nodes in the breast, or calcified fibroadenomas. This ensures that others who look at the mammogram will not misinterpret the benign finding as suspicious. This finding is recorded in the mammogram report to help when comparing to future mammograms.

Category 3: Probably benign finding – Followup in a short time frame is suggested.
The findings in this category have a very good chance (greater than 98%) of being benign (not cancer). The findings are not expected to change over time. But since it is not proven benign, it is helpful to see if an area of concern does change over time.

Follow-up with repeat imaging is usually done in 6 months and regularly thereafter until the finding is known to be stable (usually at least 2 years). This approach helps avoid unnecessary biopsies, but if the area does change over time, it allows for early diagnosis.

Category 4: Suspicious abnormality – Biopsy should be considered.
Findings do not definitely look like cancer but could be cancer. The radiologist is concerned enough to recommend a biopsy. The findings in this category can have a wide range of suspicion levels. For this reason, some doctors may divide this category further, as:

- Finding with a low suspicion of being cancer.
- Finding with an intermediate suspicion of being cancer.
- Finding of moderate concern of being cancer, but not as high as category 5.

N.B.: Not all clinicians use these subcategories.

Category 5: Highly suggestive of malignancy – Appropriate action should be taken.
The findings look like cancer and have a high chance (at least 95%) of being cancer. Biopsy is very strongly recommended.

Category 6: Known biopsy-proven malignancy – Appropriate action should be taken.
This category is used only for findings on a mammogram that have already been shown to be cancer by a previous biopsy. Mammograms may be used in this way to see how well the cancer is responding to treatment.

CRITICAL THINKING EXERCISE 8-2

United States' guidelines recommend all pregnant women be screened for HBsAg. What is the purpose of this screening? Should a woman be able to refuse screening?

BI-RADS Reporting for Breast Density

Mammogram reports can also include an assessment of breast density. BI-RADS classifies breast density into four groups:

BI-RADS 1: The breast is almost entirely fat.

This means that fibrous and glandular tissue makes up less than 25% of the breast.

BI-RADS 2: There are scattered fibroglandular densities.

Fibrous and glandular tissue makes up from 25 to 50% of the breast.

BI-RADS 3: The breast tissue is heterogeneously dense.

A&P BRAIN DRAIN BOX 8-3

What disease does the Snellen sign indicate?

The breast has more areas of fibrous and glandular tissue (from 51% to 75%) that are found throughout the breast. This can make it hard to see small masses (cysts or tumors).

BI-RADS 4: The breast tissue is extremely dense.

Diagnostic Imaging

Electroencephalograph (EEG)

Use capital letters to refer to anatomic areas and lowercase letters to refer to the positions of relative electrodes. Electrodes placed on the left use odd numbers, whereas electrodes placed on the right use even numbers. The letter *z* refers to midline (zero) electrodes. While expression of arabic numbers and lowercase letters may be subscripted, subscripting, superscripting, and various other symbols are not compatible in systems across the board, causing such items to be omitted or translated incorrectly. Therefore, the trend is for those to be expressed on the same line without subscripting.

Head Injury Imaging Reporting and Data System (HI-RADS)

HI-RADS standardizes the reporting and data collection of imaging for traumatic brain injury (TBI). It enables the radiology community to apply consistent terminology related to diagnosis of TBI, to reduce imaging interpretation variability and errors, to enhance communication with referring clinicians, and to facilitate quality assurance and research.

The American College of Radiology developed the Head Injury Institute (HII) to work on two projects related to creating standards. First, a traumatic brain injury white paper is being developed to summarize existing evidence supporting the use of different types of imaging in TBI patients in addition to formulating suitable recommendations for the same. The second project will build on the TBI Common Data Elements (CDE) developed by the National Institute of Neurological Disorders and Stroke. It will consist of an easy-to-use computer system that will allow a clinician to review a head CT or a brain MRI, and very intuitively navigate through the CDE fields to obtain a standardized report.

Liver Imaging Reporting and Data System (LI-RADS)

LI-RADS was created to standardize the reporting and data collection of CT and MR imaging for hepatocellular carcinoma (HCC). This method of categorizing liver findings for patients with cirrhosis or other risk factors for developing HCC allows the radiology community to:

- Apply consistent terminology
- Reduce imaging interpretation variability and errors
- Enhance communication with referring clinicians
- Facilitate quality assurance and research

LI-RADS currently applies to patients with cirrhosis or those at risk for HCC. HCC is cancer of the liver. The general schema of LI-RADS is to attempt to classify observations as either definite HCC (LR5) or definitely benign (LR1).

Ancillary features that may favor HCC may be applied to upgrade category by one or more categories (up to but not beyond LR4). They cannot be used to upgrade category to LR5. Absence of these features should not be used to downgrade the LR category.

Ancillary features that may favor benignity may be applied to downgrade category by one or more categories. Absence of these features should not be used to upgrade the LR category.

Electrocardiogram (ECG or EKG)

ECG and *EKG* are both acceptable abbreviations for *electrocardiogram, electrocardiographic,* and *electrocardiography*. Do not change to an abbreviation when the full term is dictated.

Use roman numerals with standard bipolar leads.

Ex: lead I, lead II, lead III

Use a lowercase *a* followed by a capital *V*, then a capital *R* (right), *L* (left), or *F* (foot) for augmented limb leads.

Ex: aVR, aVF, aVL

Use a capital *V* followed by an arabic numeral for precordial leads. While it is acceptable to subscript numbers in these expressions, subscripting, superscripting, and various other symbols are not compatible in systems across the board, causing such items to be omitted or translated incorrectly. Therefore, it is recommended to place numbers on the same line.

Ex: V1, V2, V3, V4, etc.

Expression of sequential leads uses the word *through*, not a hyphen.

Ex: leads V1 through V5 **not** V1-V5 **and not** V1-5

Magnetic Resonance Imaging (MRI)

The frequency and phase-encoding term *k-space* should be hyphenated whether used as a noun or adjective.

Relaxation times should be expressed with a *T*, arabic numbers, and lowercase letters.

X-ray

Lowercase and hyphenate *x-ray(s)* whether used as a noun, verb, or adjective. Capitalize *x-ray* only when it begins a sentence.

Use *plain*, **not** *plane*, when describing an x-ray that has been performed without contrast, as compared to an x-ray or CT scan performed with contrast. This is not referring to the directional term *plane*.

CRITICAL THINKING EXERCISE 8-3

As a medical editor working in a hospital pathology department, you notice that an acquaintance has been received into the morgue after surgery, and an autopsy is pending. The autopsy is being done without permission from the next of kin. Can an autopsy be done without permission? Explain why or why not.

Ultrasonography

A number of types of ultrasounds are performed and mentioned in dictation. Examples include abdominal ultrasound, pelvic ultrasound, transvaginal and transrectal ultrasounds, obstetric ultrasound, plus carotid and aortic ultrasounds.

Echocardiogram

An echocardiogram can use two-dimensional, three-dimensional, or Doppler ultrasound to create images of the heart. *Echocardiogram* should be transcribed when the word is dictated in full.

The brief form *echo* may be used when dictated as such, if there is no room for misinterpretation, and if the account specifics allow for the brief form to be used.

Express two-dimensional and three-dimensional with an arabic number and a capital letter *D*.

Ex: 2D echocardiogram, 3D echocardiogram

🧠 A&P BRAIN DRAIN BOX 8-4

What disease does the prayer sign indicate?

INDEX OF RADIOLOGY REPORTS

Student Name: _____   Date: _____

ID Number	Patient Name	Type of Report/Procedure
R-1	Agnes Wenceslas	CT scan of brain
R-2	Lois Jensen	Bilateral low-dose mammograms
R-3	Lois Jensen	Right breast mammogram
R-4	Christopher Lorenes	Pain management
R-5	Benjamin Helland	MRI, left knee
R-6	J. Bruce Randolph	Carotid ultrasound
R-7	Bonnie Gentry Parker	Bilateral mammograms
R-8	Yolanda Benavides	Right upper quadrant sonogram
R-9	Yolanda Benavides	Acute abdominal series
R-10	Lula Belle Shaefer	Ultrasound-guided left hip aspiration
R-11	Martha Whitsall	Whole-body bone scan
R-12	Harold Hines	CT scan of left hip
R-3401	Steve Burger	CT scan of brain without contrast
R-2558	Linda Ferguson	CT scan, abdomen/pelvis, without IV contrast
R-3770	Jackson Chandler	CT scan of the chest with contrast
R-4110	Brock J. Higgins	CT scan, soft tissues of neck, with and without contrast
R-4987	Allen Rettenbaum	CTA, chest, with contrast
R-6013	Glenn Edward Gray	CT scan of the brain without contrast
R-4334	Miguel D. Hernandez	CTA examination of neck with contrast
R-0245	Pierino Mastrone	CT, abdomen, with and without contrast
R-5037	Charles Johnson	CT angiogram, chest
R-2489	George Paul Stevens	CT, thorax, without contrast
R-0211	Jeremiah Johnson	CTA with attention to the patient's dialysis graft in the left forearm
R-0479	Julia Zapata	CT scan of the lumbar spine
R-1291	J. Edgar Rogers	CT scan, abdomen and pelvis, with oral and intravenous contrast
R-5779	Kerry Andrews	MRI of lumbar spine without contrast
R-7021	Katrina Lewis	MRI of the abdomen = MRCP
R-6890	Christopher Rackers	MRI of right knee without contrast
R-5723-a	Sandra Patterson	MRA, intracranial vessels without contrast
R-5723-b	Sandra Patterson	MRA, intracranial vessels without contrast
R-5723-c	Sandra Patterson	MRA, intracranial vessels without contrast
R-5691	Joyce A. King	MRA and MRI
R-3382	Thomas Henry Nunley	MRI, lumbar spine, with and without contrast
R-2391	Frank Samuels	MRA of head without contrast
R-3588	Andrea Nicole Scaglioni	Magnetic resonance imaging (MRI), brain
R-6437	Gene Simmons	MRI, brain, with and without contrast
R-5887	Robin Walters	MRI, left knee, without contrast
R-7754	Ernestine Tillman	MRI, lumbar spine, without contrast

R-478	Katherine Acosta	Routine bilateral screening mammograms
R-654	Carol Collins	Left mammogram, unilateral
R-371	Ann Atwell	Bilateral digital mammograms, diagnostic, with CAD and left breast ultrasound
R-525	Cathy Emmer	Bilateral digital mammograms, diagnostic, with CAD and right breast ultrasound
R-3012	Olga Ruth Smithson	Left breast needle localization procedure
R-3145	Alice Dorine McMillen	Nuclear medicine myocardial rest/stress perfusion scan
R-3057	Rose Mary Bonavia	Whole-body F-18 FDG PET/CT fusion scan
R-3092	David G. McDonald	Endoscopic retrograde ERCP
R-3145	Andrea Irene Liepold	Lumbar myelogram
R-3102	Ned G. Seferian	Myelogram of cervical spine and lumbar spine
R-3178	Carmen P. DuBose	Whole-body F-18 FDG PET/CT fusion scan
R-1103	Victor Ahearn	Injection, right knee
R-1245	Jude Milton Hale	Angiogram
R-2237	Francine Higgins	Diagnostic LP under fluoroscopic guidance
R-4025	Daniel J. Bennett	Placement of 8.5-French drain
R-8921	Miguel Trujillo	Bone marrow biopsy
R-2311	Rick Hunter	Abdominal aorta ultrasound
R-2291	P. J. Mastrone	Abdominal ultrasound
R-7384	Isabella Blanca	Ultrasound of abdomen, limited
R-3317	Saul Stuart	Renal and aortic Doppler
R-3201	Jennifer LeBlanc	Ultrasound, right breast
R-3690	Jorge Sanchez	Gallbladder ultrasound
R-2557	Mary Ellen Pollard	Renal ultrasound, limited
R-6854	Danielle J. Peterson	Pelvic ultrasound
R-7281	Jesse Garza	Ultrasound, venous Doppler, right
R-8591	Gale Lia Norton	Nuclear medicine: thyroid ultrasound
R-9065	Alice White	Nuclear medicine myocardial rest/stress perfusion scan with regional wall motion analysis and left ventricular ejection fraction calculation
R-2011	Henry Bernick	Nuclear medicine ventilation/perfusion lung scan
R-4402	Timothy Conners	Nuclear medicine hepatobiliary scan with gallbladder ejection fraction
R-4315	Susan Ziebarth	Nuclear medicine bone scan
R-5424	Olga McKeever	Nuclear medicine sentinel node injections
R-3987	George Tudor	MRI of neck/left parotid with and without gadolinium

CHAPTER 9

ACUTE CARE

LEARNING OBJECTIVES

1. How do emergency department treatment records and admission history and physical examinations differ?

2. Explain the difference between a subjective examination and an objective examination.

3. Describe the five main points necessary in a dictated operative report.

4. Explain how a hospitalist might enter into treatment for an acute care patient.

5. Define *"turn-around time"* (TAT) and list the actual times involved in this process.

6. Explain why the TAT would differ for an admission history and physical examination and for a discharge summary. How would this affect the medical editor's job?

INTRODUCTION

Acute care medical editing involves patient records dictated in a hospital or acute care setting. During a patient's admission, these reports are used to document the initial condition and symptoms, treatment, and progress or decline of a patient's status, laboratory and diagnostic studies, procedures performed, consultations with specialists, and other caregivers. These report types include but are not limited to:

Emergency department (ED) treatment records

Admitting history and physical examinations (H&Ps)

Consultations

Operative reports (OPs)

Discharge summaries (DS)

Radiology reports are dictated in hospital and acute care settings (see Chapter 8). Although pathology reports (frozen-section reports, histology, and cytology reports), death summaries, and autopsies are also documented in the hospital setting, these types of specialized reports are not included in this text.

Patients who enter the ED for treatment have a medical record created by the ED physician. This record documents all known demographic information, the reason(s) the patient came to the ED, the treatment the patient received there, plus discharge instructions or follow-up advice, as necessary. Patients who need further treatment or surgery are admitted to the hospital directly from the ED. In those cases, the ED treatment record follows the patient during the admission process and throughout the hospital stay.

After a patient is admitted to the hospital, the admitting or attending physician dictates an admitting H&P. This report includes demographics, reason(s) for admission, medical history, social and family history, and medication and allergy history. A review of systems is taken (a subjective examination), and a physical examination is performed (an objective examination). *N.B.*: Hospitalists, physicians who usually specialize in internal medicine, often dictate records for admitting physicians. This medical specialty has the responsibility of admitting patients to hospitals, making daily rounds, dictating orders, and finally discharging patients. Hospitalist groups might work on a contract basis with physician groups or with an individual physician to provide hospital coverage.

If the admitting or attending physician needs advice from a physician in a particular specialty, a consultation is requested. The consultation is dictated after the consulting physician or surgeon has made a complete examination of both the patient and the patient's records. It contains all the elements of an H&P in addition to a plan for treatment or surgery plus a prognosis.

If surgery is required on the patient, a surgeon is called in; perhaps the consulting physician is a surgeon. The surgeon will examine the patient and all the patient records, determine the best course of action, and discuss this with the patient and the patient's family, when possible. There are cases, of course, when surgery must be performed immediately after direct admission from the ED, so the discussion cannot always be held before the fact. After the surgical procedure has been completed, an operative report is dictated. This report is quite detailed, containing preoperative and postoperative diagnoses, the findings and details of procedures performed, the condition of the patient after surgery, and any postoperative advice necessary. This document must be dictated and transcribed immediately after surgery and placed on the patient's chart so that other physicians and allied health personnel can refer to it in their subsequent treatment of the patient.

When the patient recovers and is ready for discharge, the admitting or attending physician (or the hospitalist) will dictate a discharge summary (DS). This report includes some of the information contained in all of the aforementioned reports; it summarizes the patient's admission. The DS also contains the condition of the patient on discharge, medications prescribed, instructions for continued care and therapy, prognosis, and dates for follow-up office visits. These follow-up dates could include the surgeon's office and other doctor's offices or therapist's offices as well.

See the following model reports for examples of acute care reports. See Formatting Acute Care Reports on page 64 for more details.

🧠 A&P BRAIN DRAIN BOX 9-1

Name the tonsils removed most often in childhood.

⚙ CRITICAL THINKING EXERCISE 9-1

A 22-year-old Caucasian woman visits her dermatologist to have a mole on her thigh examined. The patient has a dark tan from playing volleyball with her friends on the weekends during the summer months and using a tanning bed during the winter months. The dermatologist takes a biopsy of the mole, which shows a form of skin cancer. How does this patient's history indicate her risk for skin cancer? What different types of skin cancer could this patient have? Which one(s) could be deadly? What steps can be taken to prevent skin cancer?

MODEL REPORT 1: ACUTE CARE

GENERAL SURGERY/PLASTIC SURGERY

Patient Name: Martha Ellen Smith   **ID#**: S-6
Date of Operation: 11 Jan ----   **Age/Sex**: 69/Female

PREOPERATIVE DIAGNOSIS: Right breast cancer, scheduled for bilateral mastectomies with immediate reconstruction.

POSTOPERATIVE DIAGNOSIS: Right breast cancer.

SURGEON: Danila R. Fry, MD

ASSISTANT: James A. McClure Jr, MD

ANESTHESIA: General endotracheal by Chuck Delaney, MD

OPERATIONS PERFORMED
1. Right modified radical mastectomy.
2. Left simple mastectomy.
3. Immediate bilateral breast reconstructions with tissue expanders.

MATERIAL FORWARDED TO LABORATORY FOR EXAMINATION: Mastectomy specimens.

INDICATIONS: Patient is a 69-year-old female with a previously diagnosed right breast cancer that was incompletely excised at the previous biopsy with sentinel node sampling. She was scheduled for return to the OR for completion mastectomy on the right and prophylactic mastectomy on the left. Patient desired immediate breast reconstruction. She was expected to receive no postoperative irradiation. The use of tissue expanders with subsequent implants was discussed with her as well as other options. She agreed to proceed with immediate tissue expander reconstruction. Risks and benefits were discussed. Questions were answered to the satisfaction of the patient and her husband. Informed consent was obtained to proceed.

PROCEDURE IN DETAIL: Patient was marked in the preoperative holding area. She was taken to the operating room where she was placed on the operating table in supine position. Cardiac monitors were attached, and general endotracheal anesthesia was induced. Patient's selected mastectomy incisions were demarcated on each breast to include the previous biopsy sites. Mastectomies were performed by Dr. McClure, and that portion of the case will be dictated by the general surgery service.

Once the mastectomies were completed, the plastic surgery team assumed care of the patient. The pectoralis muscle was incised along the direction of the fibers at the lateral aspect, and dissection was carried laterally beneath the serratus fascia and medially beneath the pectoralis major. Inferiorly, the pectoralis muscle was left attached to the overlying dermis. The pocket was dissected down to the level of the inframammary fold. Once an adequate pocket had been created, the tissue expander was brought

(Continued)

Patient Name: Martha Ellen Smith
Date of Operation: 11 Jan ----
ID#: S-6
Page 2

up onto the field and placed in an antibiotic irrigation solution. It was tested for manufacturing defects. None were found. It was degassed in standard fashion and filled with 50 mL of normal saline through a closed system.

The expanders were prepared and placed in identical fashion on both sides in the pockets previously created. The split pectoralis muscle was reapproximated over the implant, and total muscle coverage was achieved over both implants. A 7 mm flat Blake drain was placed along the inframammary fold and in the axillae bilaterally, then brought up through separate stab incisions in the lateral inframammary fold. They were secured in place with 3-0 nylon sutures. The wounds were copiously irrigated with normal saline, and meticulous hemostasis was assured.

Wounds were closed with interrupted 3-0 Monocryl dermal sutures followed by a running 4-0 Monocryl subcuticular suture. The ports were accessed percutaneously using the magnetic port finders included with the expanders using the supplied 23-gauge needles. Saline was immediately aspirated from both expanders. An additional 50 mL of saline was placed into each expander, and absolutely no tension was identified on the skin flaps. At the completion of the operation, the skin flaps appeared healthy to the flap margins. Drains were placed to bulb suction. Patient was extubated and transferred to the recovery room in good condition. No known complications evident at the time of this dictation.

SPONGE COUNT VERIFIED: Final correct.

DRAINS: 7 mm flat Blake x4 (two in each breast).

INTRAVENOUS FLUIDS: 3300 mL crystalloid.

ESTIMATED BLOOD LOSS: 150 mL.

URINE OUTPUT: 350 mL.

PROSTHETIC DEVICES
- Right breast: Mentor REF No. 354-6224, lot #5625290, serial #5625267-034
- Left breast: Mentor REF No. 354-6224, lot #5596178, serial #5596117-078

Danila R. Fry, MD, Plastic Surgery

DRF:xx
D: 1/11/----
T: 1/12/----

C: Jean W. Mooney, MD, Internal Medicine

MODEL REPORT 2

EMERGENCY DEPARTMENT TREATMENT RECORD

Patient Name: Roy T. Holliday   **PCP**: Unknown
Date of Exam: 11/11/----   **Age/Sex**: 14/M
ID#: M-50

CONSULTING SERVICE: Neurosurgery.

CHIEF COMPLAINT: Status post motor vehicle collision with head injury.

MODE OF ARRIVAL: Code 3, EMS.

HISTORY OF PRESENT ILLNESS: This is a 14-year-old male who was involved in an MVC. It was a vehicle versus tree. The patient was an unrestrained passenger. The patient came in after suffering a large blow to the right side of the head. EMS picked up the patient, put the patient in a C-collar, provided C-spine support, started him on some oxygen, and transferred him to the Hillcrest Medical Center Emergency Room, Code 3. The patient presented with a GCS of 4 and was posturing.

PRIMARY SURVEY
A. Airway: The patient had no spontaneous breaths.
B. Breathing: Lungs sounds were clear to auscultation with bag-valve mask.
C. Circulation: Distal pulses were 2+ in all extremities.
D. Disability: The patient had decerebrate posturing and other than posturing, did not spontaneously move extremities. GCS was 4 upon arrival.

PRIMARY INTERVENTIONS: Secondary IV access was obtained. The patient was placed on 100% oxygen with a bag-valve mask and given breaths. He was placed on a monitor. The patient was prepared for intubation. He was hyperventilated with the bag-valve mask. Patient was given 20 of etomidate and 100 of succinylcholine. The patient was intubated with RSI technique while holding C-spine precautions. A Mac 3 blade was inserted into the oropharynx. Suction was used to get out blood and debris. The vocal cords were visualized, and a 7.0 tube was passed and visualized through the vocal cords. After the tube was passed, tube placement was confirmed with bilateral breath sounds and positive color change on 6 breaths using end-tidal CO_2.

SECONDARY SURVEY: GENERAL: The patient was now GCS of 3T. His vital signs were stable. His blood pressure was 150/98 with heart rate of 100 and sinus tachycardia. He had no spontaneous breaths. Temperature was 97.1, and he was saturating 100% on monitor. He was 3T and unresponsive. HEENT: The patient had a large, 5 cm gaping laceration to the right temporoparietal area. Also in the same region, the patient had a depressed skull fracture. He had a small laceration on his chin. Patient had no hemotympanum. No septal hematoma, and his midface was stable. HEART: Regular rate and rhythm. Normal S1, S2. No murmurs, gallops, or rubs. LUNGS: Clear to auscultation bilaterally. ABDOMEN: Soft and nondistended. He had a stable chest and stable pelvis. EXTREMITIES: Two-plus pulses in all extremities. No other cyanosis, clubbing, or edema. He had no other evidence of trauma, other than trauma to the head. SKIN: No petechiae, purpura, or rashes.

(Continued)

Patient Name: Roy T. Holliday
Date of Exam: 11/11/----
ID#: M-50
Page 2

SECONDARY INTERVENTION: The patient was given 2 mg of Versed and was given 50 g of mannitol. He had an additional 2 repeat boluses of Versed. He was given 30 mg of rocuronium and another 2 mg of Versed. He was given a gram of Ancef. He was given Cerebyx 1 g.

An OG tube was placed. Placement was confirmed, and the patient's stomach was decompressed. A trauma panel was drawn and sent, and the patient was turned over to Trauma Surgery to take to the CT scanner. Also, portable chest x-ray was obtained, which showed no pneumothorax, normal mediastinum, and good tube placement.

EMERGENCY DEPARTMENT COURSE: The patient remained hemodynamically stable while in the emergency department. Patient was given therapy to help with suspected increased intracranial pressure to include mannitol and fosphenytoin. Patient was taken to CT scanner by Trauma Surgery.

IMPRESSION/MEDICAL DECISION-MAKING: This is a 14-year-old male who presents Code 3 by EMS, who has a depressed skull fracture and a large gash to his right head consistent with an open skull fracture. The patient presented with a GCS of 4, was intubated, and it was 3T upon discharge from the ED to Trauma Surgery. The patient was given 1 g Ancef to cover antibiotic wise. I suspect the patient had increased ICP based on posturing in the emergency department. He was intubated and stabilized in the ED prior to being transferred to Trauma Surgery. The blood results and CT scan to be followed by Trauma Surgery.

DISPOSITION: Admission to the SICU in critical condition.

EMERGENCY DEPARTMENT DIAGNOSES
1. Depressed skull fracture.
2. Blunt head injury.
3. Status post motor vehicle collision.

PROGNOSIS: Guarded.

_____
Samuel Ernest, MD, Emergency Department

SE:xx
D: 11/11/----
T: 11/11/----

c: Arnold R. Youngblood, MD, Neurosurgery
   Mack Stolga, MD, Trauma Surgery

MODEL REPORT 3

ORTHOPEDIC SURGERY

Patient Name: Mary Jane Alderman   **ID#**: S-12
Date of Operation: 23 Feb ----   **Age/Sex**: 45/F

PREOPERATIVE DIAGNOSIS: Left shoulder impingement syndrome.

POSTOPERATIVE DIAGNOSIS: Left shoulder impingement syndrome.

SURGEON: Raj Patel, MD

ASSISTANT: Jack Zullig, MD

ANESTHESIA: General endotracheal by Carl Erickson Avalon, MD

OPERATIONS PERFORMED
1. Examination under anesthesia.
2. Left shoulder diagnostic arthroscopy.
3. Subacromial decompression.
4. Distal clavicle revision.

SPECIMEN REMOVED: None.

INDICATIONS: This is a 45-year-old female with left shoulder impingement. She is right-hand dominant. She has no history of trauma. The patient has painful and limited range of motion. The patient also has acromioclavicular joint arthritis. The patient had workup done consisting of plain films and MRI, which showed a possible fear of the supraspinatus and possible labral pathology. Acromioclavicular joint arthrosis.

FINDINGS: Diffuse synovitis in the patient's left shoulder. The synovitis does not extend into the biceps. The patient has the labrum intact. There is some fraying anteriorly. No loose bodies in the patient's glenohumeral joint. The patient has no rotator cuff pathology.

PROCEDURE IN DETAIL: During the preoperative visit, the patient's diagnosis, risks, benefits, and adverse effects were discussed with the patient by Dr. Craven. All questions were answered. Informed written and verbal consent were obtained.

On the day of surgery, patient was brought to the anesthesia holding area. The operative surgeon identified and marked the appropriate surgical site. The operative nurse and anesthesia team evaluated the patient. The patient was brought back to the operating suite and transferred to the operating table. She was given preoperative antibiotics by Anesthesia. She was then given general endotracheal anesthesia by Anesthesia. The patient was positioned appropriately on the beach chair.

(Continued)

Patient Name: Mary Jane Alderman
Date of Operation: 23 Feb ----
ID#: S-12
Page 2

The patient's left shoulder was examined under anesthesia. She has symmetric passive range of motion compared to the opposite side except for external rotation. With the elbows abducted approximately 90 degrees, the patient has approximately 10 degrees' decrease in external rotation in the left shoulder compared to the right shoulder. Forward flexion and abduction were symmetric to the opposite side, otherwise. Given that the patient's external rotation with the arm at 80 to 90 degrees was decreased, gentle manipulation was done to help release part of that.

The patient's left shoulder was then prepped and draped in the usual sterile fashion. Diagnostic arthroscopy was begun with placing a portal superiorly in the standard fashion. Prior to portal placement, the acromion AC anatomic landmarks were drawn out with a marking pen. A posterior portal approximately 2 fingerbreadths below and 1 fingerbreadth medial to the posterolateral corner of the acromion was made. This was initially done by injecting 60 mL of fluid into the AC joint. Once the AC joint was distended, next a skin incision was made with an 11 blade. A trocar was then inserted into the joint. Fluid was seen coming out through the trocar; therefore, it was known that we were in the joint. Next a scope was placed through the posterior portal. A diagnostic arthroscopy was begun. The patient was found to have significant synovitis.

Next, under direct visualization an anterior portal was made. This was done by splitting the distance between the coracoid and the anterolateral edge of the acromion. An 18-gauge needle was used. As stated, this was made under direct visualization. Once this portal was made, a yellow trocar was placed into the portal site. A probe was then inserted through this portal, and the diagnostic arthroscopy was begun.

The biceps tendon was visualized. It appeared to be intact. There was noted to be significant synovitis. The inferior and superior edges of the labrum were probed and noted to be intact. The patient's inferior recess had no evidence of loose bodies. The patient's rotator cuff was then evaluated and appeared to be intact. Some mild debridement at the synovium was done with a 4.5 shaver.

Next, attention was turned to the subacromial decompression. The posterior trocar was removed. It was reinserted into the subacromial space. A lateral portal was then made. This was to get into the subacromial space. Once the lateral portal was made, a 4.5 shaver was placed into the subacromial space. The subacromial bursa was debrided. Once adequate debridement had been done, anatomic landmarks inside the joint were identified at the anterolateral corner, the posterolateral corner, and the AP joint. These were visualized. Next an ArthroWand was used to help debride some of the soft tissue. Next a bur was used to do the acromioplasty. The acromioplasty was started at the anterolateral portion, then progressed medially. Once it was determined that an adequate acromioplasty had been done, the attention was then turned to the clavicle.

(Continued)

Patient Name: Mary Jane Alderman
Date of Operation: 23 Feb ----
ID#: S-12
Page 3

A distal clavicle incision was done arthroscopically. The distal clavicle joint was identified. Using both the 4.5 shaver and the ArthroWand, the soft tissue was debrided. Next, through the anterior portal the bur was reinserted, and the distal clavicle excision was made. Once it was thought that adequate resection of the distal clavicle had been done, the bur was removed. The anterior incision was slightly extended. Fingertip was used to palpate the acromioclavicular joint. A cross-arm test was done to see if further resection needed to be done. It was determined that more distal clavicle needed to be excised.

Once again the bur was placed through the anterior portal, and more of the distal clavicle was excised. Approximately 1 cm of the distal clavicle was excised. Next the bur was removed. Again the cross-arm test was done, and there was noted no abutment from the distal clavicle and the acromion. Once all this had been completed, the instruments were removed from the shoulder.

The skin was reapproximated anteriorly, since the portal was extended, with horizontal mattress using 3-0 nylon. Arthroscopic portals were closed with a port stitch using 3-0 nylon. Xeroform and a sterile dressing were applied. Sterile dressing consisted of flats and an ABD, both in the axilla and on top of the wound. Hypafix tape was then applied. We injected 40 mg of methylprednisolone and Marcaine into the joint prior to putting on the sterile dressing. The patient tolerated the procedure well and was aroused from her general endotracheal anesthesia.

INTRAVENOUS FLUIDS: 140 mL lactated Ringer's.

ESTIMATED BLOOD LOSS: Less than 10 mL.

TOURNIQUET TIME: Not used.

DISPOSITION: Patient will be taken to the PACU for recovery, then discharged to follow up. Patient is scheduled for physical therapy appointment on 26 Feb, Monday, at 0830 hours. She will be given proper handouts and directions.

_____

Raj Patel, MD, Orthopedic Surgery

RP:xx
D: 2/23/----
T: 2/24/----

c: Margaret Craven, MD, Orthopedic Shoulder Specialist

MODEL REPORT 4

OPHTHALMOLOGIC SURGERY

Patient Name: Mario Bozzi   **ID#**: S-20
Date of Operation: 11 July ----   **Age/Sex**: 59/Male

PREOPERATIVE DIAGNOSIS: Temporal arteritis.

POSTOPERATIVE DIAGNOSIS: Temporal arteritis.

SURGEON: Yasmin Naimi, MD

ASSISTANT: Jimmy Dale Jett, RN, Circulating Nurse

ANESTHESIA: Local MAC by Chuck Delaney, MD

OPERATION PERFORMED: Biopsy of left temporal artery.

MATERIAL FORWARDED TO LABORATORY FOR EXAMINATION: Portion of temporal artery.

PROCEDURE IN DETAIL: After having been properly identified in the preop holding area, the patient was brought to OR 3 and placed under monitored anesthesia control (MAC). At this point a Doppler ultrasound was used to trace the course of the left temporal artery, and a surgical marking pen was used to outline this course.

The temple area was shaved using a standard disposable razor. The skin was then prepped with 5% povidone-iodine and draped in the usual sterile fashion to isolate the left temporal artery. After prepping, local anesthesia consisting of 2% lidocaine with epinephrine was slowly injected through a 25-gauge needle parallel to the artery.

Next, gentle traction was used to pull the skin taut as a #15 blade was used to bisect the skin adjacent to the underlying artery. Small mosquito forceps was used to dissect toward the temporal artery in a subcutaneous plane, at which point the temporal artery was identified. Careful blunt dissection along the side of the vessel was used to expose the artery.

At this point, 4-0 silk sutures were used to ligate the exposed temporal artery, 2 sutures on either end, both the proximal and distal ends of the temporal artery. Two small feeder vessels were also ligated using a single 4-0 silk suture.

Next, suture scissors were used to cut the temporal artery in between the distal and proximal ends, where the sutures had been previously placed to ligate the artery. After the artery had been removed, it was measured and determined to be 2.5 cm. It was then placed in formalin for pathologic inspection. General cautery was used to control areas of residual bleeding.

(Continued)

Patient Name: Mario Bozzi
Date of Operation: 11 July ----
ID#: S-20
Page 2

Next, two 6-0 Vicryl sutures were used to close the subcutaneous tissue layer. Finally, skin closure was obtained by placing six 6-0 fast-absorbing gut sutures. Bacitracin ophthalmic ointment was applied to the wound, and a 2 × 2 gauze sponge was placed lengthwise over the wound, and a Tegaderm tape was placed over this gauze.

The patient was returned to the postoperative recovery room in stable condition.

FLUIDS: None.

ESTIMATED BLOOD LOSS: Minimal.

COMPLICATIONS: None.

DISPOSITION: Stable.

_____

Yasmin Naimi, MD, Ophthalmology

YN:xx
D: 7/11/----
T: 7/12/----

c: Jean W. Mooney, MD, Internal Medicine

MODEL REPORT 5

GENITOURINARY SURGERY

Patient Name: Tuong Van Nguyen   **ID#**: S-63
Date of Operation: 04/20/----   **Age/Sex**: 51/M

PREOPERATIVE DIAGNOSIS: Bilateral ureteral obstruction from recurrent retroperitoneal fibrosis.

POSTOPERATIVE DIAGNOSIS: Recurrent retroperitoneal fibrosis with bilateral ureteral obstructions.

OPERATIONS PERFORMED
1. Bilateral ureteral lyses.
2. Left ureteral resection.
3. Left ileal ureter interposition.
4. Right omental flap.

SPECIMENS REMOVED
1. Left ureter.
2. Right retroperitoneal biopsy.

SURGEON: Charles Mendesz, MD

FIRST ASSISTANT: Ken Miller, MD

SECOND ASSISTANT: Jimmy Dale Jett, RN

ANESTHETIC: General with epidural regional block by Carl Erickson Avalon, MD

DRAINS: 10 mm flat Jackson-Pratt, left lower quadrant; 20-French Foley catheter in bladder; nasogastric tube.

SPONGE COUNT: Verified x3.

PROSTHETIC DEVICES: None.

INDICATIONS: This is a 51-year-old Vietnamese male with a history of retroperitoneal fibrosis who underwent a laparoscopic bilateral ureterolysis 2 years ago, after which he did well until early this year when on surveillance it was noted that his creatinine had increased from 1.1 to 1.8. Cystoscopy, retrograde pyelograms, and stent placements were performed in February of this year. His creatinine level returned to normal. Followup CT scanning demonstrated recurrent retroperitoneal fibrosis, which had extended down into his midureters previously. The obstruction was at the level of the proximal ureters. Patient was informed of his options for treatment to include medical treatment alone, surgical treatment alone, and combination therapy. Indwelling ureteral stents were also offered. He has had significant side effects from the ureteral stents, and he decided to be stent-free. After an extended consultation with the patient, it was decided that his best chance for long-term success is to undergo repeat ureterolysis in an open fashion,

(Continued)

then have medical therapy postoperatively. In this regard, postop consultation with Rheumatology has already been arranged. Patient was informed of the indications, risks, benefits, and alternatives of the ureterolysis and possible need for ileal ureter interposition. He desired to proceed with the operation and was consented and scheduled as such.

DESCRIPTION OF OPERATION: Patient was taken to the operating room where an epidural catheter was placed by the anesthesia team. He was then placed in the supine position. General anesthetic was administered. He was prepped and draped in the usual sterile fashion. A 20-French Foley catheter was placed into his bladder on the field and damped to the drapes. A midline laparotomy incision was made from the xiphoid process lo near the pubic symphysis. Bovie electrocautery was continued down to the fascia. He had a lot of venous collaterals that required coagulation. Of note, on his preoperative imaging, he has an occluded vena cava from the retroperitoneal fibrosis.

We incised to his anterior abdominal wall fascia, sharply incised his peritoneum, and entered his abdomen. Cautery was used to incise the transversalis fascia and peritoneum. Initially we noticed not a great deal of intraabdominal adhesions noted from his previous laparoscopic procedure. The urachal remnant was isolated from his anterior abdominal wall, cut, and incised to allow better mobilization of the bladder. The Bookwalter retractor set was assembled over the wound and used for retraction as needed throughout the case.

We turned our attention first to identifying his right ureter. The right colon was reflected medially off the kidney. A great deal of adhesions were reflecting the colon off his retroperitoneum. Again, a lot of venous collaterals were noted, but hemostasis was adequate. Sharp and blunt dissection was used. We eventually found the right ureter as it crossed the pelvic brim. It was adhesiolysed from a dense, rock-hard, fibrotic mass surrounding the ureter. This was particularly evident at the pelvic brim and crossing down into the true pelvis.

Several centimeters into the true pelvis, the ureter became normal again and was easily mobilized in its most distal extent toward the bladder. Once the ureter was completely mobilized up toward the renal pelvis, an inspection of the ureter demonstrated what appeared to be an otherwise viable ureter. There was about a 1 cm segment that was perhaps slightly ischemic, but it was felt that it would probably be viable, especially given our plans for an omental wrap. We sharply excised a small portion of the fibrotic mass near the portion of the ureter that was most encased and sent this for permanent pathologic examination as a right retroperitoneal biopsy.

We then turned our attention to the left side. Of note, on his previous surgery, the left ureter was apparently placed outside the retroperitoneum by tacking the left colonic mesentery underneath the ureter. In the process of reflecting the left colon, again we

(Continued)

Patient Name: Tuong Van Nguyen
Date of Operation: 04/20/----
ID#: S-63
Page 3

found dense adhesions. We did, in fact, find the left ureter to be tented up over the left colonic mesentery in an intraabdominal fashion. We completely mobilized the ureter from the mesentery and reflected the mesentery back medially in its normal anatomic location. We mobilized the left ureter with great difficulty down to the pelvic brim. At this point, however, it was completely adherent to the surrounding retroperitoneal mass. Furthermore, the part of the ureter that was draped over the colon appeared severely ischemic and nonviable. For this reason, it was decided to incise the ureter at the level of the pelvic brim. This was done sharply, such that the previous indwelling ureteral stent could be removed intact. This was, in fact, done. With the ureter incised, we then mobilized it proximally until the ureter appeared pink and viable. It appeared viable no more than 2 to 3 cm away from the renal pelvis. When we found what appeared to be viable ureter, we excised the nonviable portion of the ureter and sent it for permanent pathology examination. In doing so, we had a gap of approximately 15 to 20 cm that needed to be bridged. We decided that ileal ureter interposition would be required on this side. We mobilized the bladder on both the left and right sides slightly; however, neither bladder pedicle required ligating. This allowed the bladder to be lifted just to the level of the pelvic brim, slightly beyond the level of the previously incised ureter on the left side.

We turned our attention to the bowel. Some adhesiolysis was required around the terminal ileum and ileocecal valve in order to properly identify the ileocecal valve. Approximately 20 cm proximal to this, we marked the distal end of our bowel segment and went about another 15 to 20 cm proximal and marked the most proximal end of our bowel segment. We ensured that the mesenteric vascular pedicle of this segment would be adequate to maintain viability of the excised ileal segment. This proved to be the case. We marked the peritoneum overlying the mesentery with Bovie electrocautery, then incised and ligated the small mesenteric vessels with interrupted silk sutures. This was done on both the proximal and distal extents. The GIA stapler was passed through the incised mesentery, completing the bowel resection proximally and distally.

We then returned bowel continuity by approximating the butt ends of the more distal ileum, excising the tips and passing the GIA 75 stapler into the bowel lumen, then firing the stapler, ensuring that the bowel was anastomosed in a side-to-side fashion with the one antimesenteric border approximating the other antimesenteric border. The GIA stapler was removed. The butt ends of the bowel anastomosis were closed with the TA 55 stapler, which was also fired without difficulty. The crotch of the anastomosis was secured with 3-0 silk sutures, and Lemberts on the butt end of the anastomosis were used to bury the staple line.

We then turned our attention to the isolated portion of ileum, which would be used for the ileoureter. We attempted to mobilize the left colonic mesentery enough to pass the ileum through a hole in the mesentery so that it would be able to lie in a retroperitoneal fashion; however, due to his retroperitoneal fibrosis, his left colonic mesentery had been sucked into the fibrotic mass somewhat, and it was very short.

(Continued)

It did not allow adequate mobility for the ileal segment to pass. We decided to drape the ileal segment over the top of the left colon. In doing so, it appeared to have more than adequate length to reach both the bladder and the incised ureter up near the left ureteropelvic junction. It also did not seem to impinge upon the left colon, such that we felt that it would function normally and be at low risk for obstruction.

With the ileal segment isolated and placed in a proper position, we first turned our attention to the proximal anastomosis. We made an approximately 1 cm incision in the proximal butt end of the ileal segment and in an end-to-side fashion anastomosed the ileum to the left proximal-most ureter. Prior to doing so, the ureter was spatulated widely. After spatulation, we passed Van Buren sounds through the ureter into the left renal pelvis to calibrate the remaining lumen, and this calibrated up to 20-French easily. He was also given an ampule of intravenous indigo carmine, and there was seen to be blue efflux from the proximal end of the ureter. Interrupted 5-0 Vicryl sutures were used to make the anastomosis between the ileum and proximal ureter. Approximately 8 to 10 anastomotic sutures were placed circumferentially in a clockwise fashion through full-thickness ureter and full-thickness bowel from mucosa to serosa. Once approximately 180 degrees of the anastomosis was completed, we opened the distal end of the ileal segment, passed a right angle through the distal end up through and into the anastomosis, grasped a 0.035-inch floppy-tipped guide wire, retracted it back through the distal end of the ileum, and then placed the proximal end into the right renal pelvis. Over this a 6-French x 30 cm double-J ureteral stent was passed through the ileum across the anastomosis and into the left renal pelvis. The wire was subsequently removed, allowing good stent placement across the proximal anastomosis with the distal end exiting the butt end of the ileal segment. The anastomosis was completed with the 5-0 Vicryl sutures proximally. It appeared to be watertight.

We then turned our attention to the distal end. The dome of the bladder was identified. The peritoneum overlying the dome was incised. The perivesicular fat was divided. Detrusor was identified, and 2-0 Vicryl stay sutures were placed on either side of the expected location of the anastomosis. The bladder was incised with Bovie electrocautery to a lumen that approximated the luminal size of the small bowel. Approximately 180 degrees of the anastomosis were again made with full-thickness bites, including the bladder mucosa and detrusor in both the serosa and mucosa of the small bowel. This was done with 3-0 Vicryl interrupted sutures. Once approximately 180 degrees of it had been completed, the distal tail of the double-J stent was placed inside the bladder, and the anastomosis was completed with interrupted sutures in 360 degrees. A second layer of closure was completed by closing the serosa and peritoneum overlying the bladder to the serosa of the small bowel with interrupted 3-0 Vicryl sutures. Again, this portion of the anastomosis appeared to be watertight. We copiously irrigated his abdomen at this point. Hemostasis appeared to be adequate. We closed the small bowel mesentery from the previous bowel resection with interrupted silk sutures, then secured the bowel anastomosis to the root of the ileal

(Continued)

Patient Name: Tuong Van Nguyen
Date of Operation: 04/20/----
ID#: S-63
Page 5

ureter mesentery, and closed any surrounding mesenteric defects with interrupted silk sutures. This included the defect that occurred where the ileal ureter passed over the top of the left colon.

We then turned our attention to wrapping the right ureter with an omental wrap. We split the patient's omentum in the midline up to the transverse colon and mobilized a portion of this omentum off the transverse colon to allow a tongue that would reach deeply into his pelvis, passing behind the right colon. In doing so, we were allowed to have piece of omentum that wrapped circumferentially around the lysed portion of the ureter circumferentially. The omentum extended down to normal distal ureter. With the omentum wrapped 350 degrees around the ureter at the level of the fibrotic mass, we secured it there with interrupted Vicryl sutures. We quickly ran his small bowel and identified no injuries. Earlier in the case, in mobilizing his right colon, there was a partial deserosalization of the cecum. This was repaired with interrupted silk Lembert sutures. Inspection of this at the conclusion of the case demonstrated an intact repair. A #10 mm flat Jackson-Pratt drain was brought into the abdomen through the left lower quadrant and was placed along the left colonic gutter near the left ileal ureter. The abdomen was subsequently closed with #1 looped PDS up to the level near the xiphoid process. Interrupted #1 Vicryl suture closed the most proximal extent of this incision near the xiphoid and allowed us to bury the knot from the PDS suture. Once all these sutures were tied and cut, his wound was copiously irrigated. Hemostasis in the superficial tissues was assured, and the skin was approximated with stainless steel staples. Sterile dressing was applied. His Jackson-Pratt drain was hooked up and secured.

Patient tolerated the procedure well, was extubated in the operating room, then taken to SICU in stable condition. He received 1250 mL of colloid and 9000 mL crystalloid. Estimated blood loss 900 mL. Urine output 1200 mL. Gastric output was 50 mL.

It should be noted that the nasogastric tube that had been placed at the start of the case was left indwelling at the conclusion of the case. It was verified in good position prior to closure.

_____

Charles Mendesz, MD, Urology

CM:xx
D: 04/21/----
T: 04/22/----

cc: Luke Mosbacker, MD, Rheumatology
    Ken Miller, MD, Gastroenterology

MODEL REPORT 6

EMERGENCY DEPARTMENT TREATMENT RECORD

Patient Name: Paula K. Lockhart   **PCP**: Linda L. Kingston, FNP
Date of Exam: 21 Oct ----   **Age/Sex**: 68-year-old female
ID#: M-52

CHIEF COMPLAINT: Left forearm pain and deformity after a fall.

MODE OF ARRIVAL: The patient arrived by privately owned vehicle.

CONSULTING SERVICE: Orthopedic Surgery.

HISTORY OF PRESENT ILLNESS: The patient is a 68-year-old female who
presents to the emergency department, accompanied by her daughter, after falling
and sustaining an injury to her left arm. The patient as well as the daughter, who was
present at the time, state that she was standing, bending over on an uneven surface,
slipped, and fell backward. She placed her arms up behind her to stop her and thus
sustained injury. There is clearly no history of loss of consciousness either before or
after the fall. No dizziness, headaches, weakness, numbness, chest pain, difficulty
breathing, or other complaints at this time. She does complain that the arm is mildly
tender to palpation. She seems to have minimal pain when the arm is not being
manipulated. She does not complain of a headache or pain to her cervical spine,
thoracic spine, or lumbar spine. There is no pain in her coccyx.

REVIEW OF SYSTEMS: The patient has a chronic cough. Her review of systems is
otherwise negative, except for the history of present illness.

PAST MEDICAL HISTORY: Hypertension.

MEDICATIONS: Please see the handwritten chart for a list of the medications.

SOCIAL HISTORY: Please see the handwritten chart for the social history.

PHYSICAL EXAMINATION: VITAL SIGNS ON PRESENTATION: Temperature of
100.2 degrees, a pulse of 88, respirations of 20, blood pressure of 170/85, oxygen
saturation 94% on room air. GENERAL APPEARANCE: That of a well-developed, well-
nourished white female in no acute distress. HEENT EXAMINATION: The pupils
are equal, round, and reactive to light. Conjunctivae are normal. The sclerae are
anicteric. The oropharynx is clear, moist, and symmetric. The nose is normal. NECK
EXAM: The neck is supple without masses. The thyroid is normal. RESPIRATORY
EXAM: The lungs are clear to auscultation bilaterally. CHEST WALL EXAM: Nontender.
CARDIOVASCULAR EXAM: SI and S2 are normal. There are no murmurs noted. There is
no peripheral edema. GASTROINTESTINAL EXAM: Abdomen is soft and nontender. No
hepatosplenomegaly is noted. INTEGUMENTARY EXAM: There are no rashes, lesions,
ulcers, or induration. NEUROLOGIC EXAM: The patient is alert and appropriate.
The speech is clear. The gait is stable. EXTREMITIES: There is some deformity over
the ulnar aspect of the forearm on the left side. There is ecchymosis noted as well.

(Continued)

Patient Name: Paula K. Lockhart
Date of Exam: 21 Oct ----
ID#: M-52
Page 2

Minimal tenderness to palpation. The anatomic snuffbox is completely nontender. The thumb and indeed the entire forearm are totally nontender with axial loading. She is neurovascularly intact. She does have some pain with extension of the wrist against resistance.

ANCILLARY STUDIES: The x-ray shows a slightly impacted but otherwise nondisplaced intraarticular distal radius fracture.

MEDICAL DECISION-MAKING PROCESS: There is an isolated distal radius fracture in an elderly female. She has very minimal pain. She is tolerating the injury quite well. Neurovascularly she is intact. Orthopedics was called down and, with some minimal intravenous narcotics, they were able to reduce and cast the fracture with the assistance of the finger traps. The patient tolerated this well.

EMERGENCY DEPARTMENT DIAGNOSIS: Distal radius fracture.

CONDITION: Stable.

DISPOSITION: The patient was discharged from the emergency department to home.

DISCHARGE INSTRUCTIONS: The patient has been discharged with clear return instructions as well as instructions to follow up at the orthopedic clinic as directed by the orthopedic team.

_____

Raj Pavari, MD, Orthopedic Surgery

RP:xx
D: 10/21/----
T: 10/21/----

C: Linda L. Kingston, FNP

MODEL REPORT 7

GASTROENTEROLOGY SURGERY

Patient Name: Charisse Moore   **ID#**: S-67
Date of Operation: 06/22/----   **Age/Sex**: 21/F

PREPROCEDURE DIAGNOSES: Acute left lower quadrant abdominal pain and peritonitis.

POSTPROCEDURE DIAGNOSES: Colonic edema, gastritis, gastric polyp.

PROCEDURES PERFORMED
1. Esophagogastroduodenoscopy.
2. Colonoscopy.

SPECIMENS REMOVED
1. Distal esophagus.
2. Antrum.
3. Gastric polyp.
4. Second portion of duodenum.
5. Surveillance biopsies, colon.

PROCEDURES PERFORMED BY: James A. McClure Jr, MD

ANESTHETIC: Propofol.

INDICATIONS: This is a 21-year-old female with a history of Wilms tumor, status post right nephrectomy, and total abdominal radiation therapy as a young child. She has a history of several years of abdominal pain. She presented acutely with onset of left lower quadrant abdominal pain 4 days prior to this procedure. She had had a history of fever prior to admission. She was found on CT scan to have diffuse bowel wall thickening as well as ascites. Her ascitic fluid was drained by Interventional Radiology 1 day prior to this procedure, and it appears to be infected with neutrophil counts greater than 5000. She has been on antibiotics for 4 days. The concern was, given her abdominal radiation, whether she had an area of ischemia, small area of volvulus, or colitis that was contributing to the onset of peritonitis. Patient does have a history of chronic recurring ascites, likely from destruction of lymph tissue from previous radiation therapy. She has been occult-blood positive while in the hospital. Stools cultured no growth at the time of endoscopy. Fecal leukocytes were zero at the time of endoscopy. She underwent the procedure given concern for significantly inflamed colon and risk of perforation.

FINDINGS
1. Esophagus: The esophagus was normal in appearance. There was no evidence of esophagitis, extrinsic mass, compression, varices, erosions, or other abnormalities. Photo documentation was obtained. Biopsies were obtained from the distal esophagus.

(Continued)

Patient Name: Charisse Moore
Date of Operation: 06/22/----
ID#: S-67
Page 2

2. Stomach: The stomach had a hypertrophic mucosal appearance, which was evidenced by scattered erythema. The gastric mucosa was easily friable with biopsy as well as with passage of the scope. No discrete ulcerations or varices were noted. A small gastric polyp approximately 0.5 cm in diameter was noted along the greater curvature of the stomach. This was isolated in appearance. Pylorus appeared normal. Photo documentation of all the above was obtained. Biopsies were obtained in the antrum as well as of the gastric polyp. They were sent to pathology for evaluation.

3. Duodenum: The duodenum was normal in appearance. No evidence of duodenitis, ulcers, nodules, polyps, masses, or vascular malformation was seen. Photo documentation of the duodenum was obtained. Biopsies were obtained from the second portion of the duodenum.

4. Colon: The visualized colonic segments were all abnormal in appearance. The mucosal surface of the colon appeared edematous with loss of vascular markings as well as crypt hyperplasia. No true structures were identified; however, segments of the colon appeared to be less distensible than others. There were no polyps, ulcers, or masses identified on examination. No areas of ischemia were noted. The colonic mucosa did appear to be slightly friable throughout. Photo documentation of colonic segments was obtained. Surveillance biopsies were obtained throughout the entirety of the colon.

DESCRIPTION OF PROCEDURE: H&P was performed prior to the procedure. Before the patient was taken from the floor, the procedure indications, potential complications, and alternatives available were explained to the patient and her mother, who was present. Patient has been on Dilaudid for pain control. Because of this, Mother co-signed the consent forms even though the patient is older than 18 years. Opportunities for questions were provided, and informed consent was obtained prior to the procedure.

In the procedural room, Betadine diluted with saline was administered via 3-way Foley intrarectally. The patient had a total of 1000 mL administered prior to the procedure in order to clear out remaining stool. Patient had been n.p.o. for 6 days prior to the procedure. Scant clots of greenish stool were noted to come out of the 3-way Foley after administration of only 250 mL of diluted Betadine; thus, the full 1000 mL was administered. Stools became clear after administration of an additional 750 mL of diluted Betadine. After this preparation enema and after sedation in the OR, an upper endoscope was passed through the incisural orifice into the oral cavity. Under direct visualization, the esophagus was intubated. The endoscope was passed down the esophagus through the stomach and into the duodenum. Careful inspection was made as the endoscope was advanced and withdrawn.

After the upper endoscope was removed, a colonoscope was inserted into the rectum, and under direct visualization it was advanced to the cecum. The terminal ileum was

(Continued)

Patient Name: Charisse Moore
Date of Operation: 06/22/----
ID#: S-67
Page 3

unable to be intubated. Careful inspection was made as the colonoscope was inserted as well as withdrawn. The quality of the preparation was good, allowing visualization of all mucosal surfaces. The patient tolerated the procedure well, and there were no complications.

RECOMMENDATIONS
1. Follow up with pathology for results of biopsies.
2. Continue Dilaudid for pain control.
3. Continue Timentin for antibiotic of choice for infected peritoneal fluid.
4. Follow up with lab for culture results, when available.
5. Encourage p.o.intake.
6. Continue total parenteral nutrition for now.
7. Patient has a PICC line in place for administration of antibiotics and TPN. Continue to monitor for clinical signs of sepsis, fever, or other bacterial infections in the line.
8. Patient to have flat and abdominal upright films after colonoscopy to allow free air, although there was no suggestion of perforation on either colonoscopic or clinical exam after the procedure.

_____
James A. McClure, MD, General Surgery

JAM:xx
D: 06/22/----
T: 06/23/----

c: Trevor Jordan, MD, Nephrology
   Sherman Loyd, MD, Internal Medicine

MODEL REPORT 8

NEPHROLOGY SURGERY

Patient Name: Amber K. Welch   **ID#**: S-94
Date of Operation: 09/16/----   **Age/Sex**: 36/F

PREOPERATIVE DIAGNOSIS: Right ureteropelvic junction obstruction with renal stones.

POSTOPERATIVE DIAGNOSIS: Right ureteropelvic junction obstruction with renal stones.

OPERATIONS PERFORMED
1. Right laparoscopic dismembered pyeloplasty.
2. Nephroscopic extraction of kidney stones.
3. Placement of ureteral stent.

SPECIMENS REMOVED: Kidney stones.

SURGEON: Charles Mendesz, MD

ASSISTANT: Trevor Jordan, MD

ANESTHETIC: General endotracheal tube by Chuck Delaney, MD

DESCRIPTION OF OPERATION: After the patient was correctly identified and informed consent was obtained, she was taken to the operating room, where she was given a general endotracheal tube anesthetic. A Foley catheter was placed in the urinary bladder, and patient was placed in a right modified lateral position. All pressure points were carefully checked and padded. Next she had a Veress needle inserted at the umbilicus, and its correct position was determined by drip test. Once the needle was found to be in the correct position, the abdomen was insufflated to 20 mmHg pressure. The abdomen was entered under directed vision using a Visiport device. There was no evidence of adhesions and no intraabdominal pathology.

A 10 mm trocar was placed midway between the umbilicus and the xiphoid process, and a 5 mm trocar placed in line with the umbilicus lateral to the rectus muscle. Using bipolar cautery, the colon was incised at the white line of Toldt and reflected medially. The ureter was identified along with a large gonadal vessel, which was somewhat adherent to the ureter. The gonadal vessel was divided to prevent shearing at the entry of the vena cava. The ureter was then completely mobilized, and there was no evidence of a lower pole crossing vessel. It appeared to be an intrinsic defect of the ureter with somewhat of a high insertion.

The ureter was then transected at the level of the ureteropelvic junction. The obstructing segment was removed. The ureter was spatulated for 1.5 cm. Then a reduction pyeloplasty was performed. Using the apex of the most dependent portion of the pelvis and the apex of the spatulated incision, the ureter was reapproximated back

(Continued)

Patient Name: Amber K. Welch
Date of Operation: 09/16/----
ID#: S-94
Page 2

to the renal pelvis. There was no significant tension whatsoever to return the ureter back to the renal pelvis. A urologic wire was placed through a trocar and down the ureter into the bladder, over which a 28 cm 7-French, double-J stent was passed. Then the wire was removed. The upper portion of the stent was placed in the upper pole of the kidney.

A flexible cystoscope was then inserted through the open renal pelvis. After vigorous irrigation, the kidney stones, which had previously been identified, were flushed out. These were removed and sent for permanent evaluation. They appeared to be calcium oxalate stones. Using the flexible cystoscope, each calyx was inspected, and we were unable to find other stones. Using 4-0 PDS suture in a running fashion, the anterior portion of the anastomosis was performed. Then the posterior portion of the anastomosis was performed. This led to some of the renal pelvis that needed to be closed. This was closed using a running 4-0 PDS suture.

Next the patient had 5 mL of Hemaseel placed over the area of the repair. A 4 mm Jackson-Pratt drain was placed through a separate stab incision in the retroperitoneum and placed overlying the area of the anastomosis. The colon was then reflected back to its usual position and tacked using a hernia tacker. Patient was awakened, extubated, and transported to the recovery room awake and in stable condition. There were no complications. The patient tolerated the procedure well. There was minimal blood loss.

_____

Charles Mendesz, MD, Nephrology

CM:xx
D: 09/16/----
T: 09/17/----

STYLES AND STANDARDS

Acute care reports are formatted much the same as the report styles mentioned in the previous Unit 4 chapters, the differences being the variations in elements and headings included. The styles outlined contain common content and headings, but it is important to remember that standardized formats and styles are currently being developed to facilitate interoperability in electronic health records.

Some of the healthcare organizations involved with standardization of medical documentation include the American Society for Testing and Materials (ASTM), the Association for Healthcare Documentation Integrity (AHDI), Health Level Seven (HL7), and Health Story Project (HSP), which is now under the management of the Health Information Management Systems Society (HIMSS). (See Appendix G for more information about these organizations.)

A&P BRAIN DRAIN BOX 9-2

List the four stages of mitosis.

Turn-Around Times

The Book of Style for Medical Transcription, 3rd edition, notes: "Turn-around time (TAT) in transcription refers to the window of time between the dictation of a report and when it is transcribed and returned to the author for authentication. This includes the period of time the report is pending transcription on the dictation system, the time it is checked out or routed to the transcriptionist, the time it is checked out or routed to a QA coordinator or editor, and any other time or delay between dictation and delivery to the author or facility."

Patient care reports serve a number of purposes during the course of a patient's treatment. TAT of these reports is a critical contributor that affects medical decision making that directly influences patient outcomes. These reports chronicle the patient's story and the reasons surrounding the events of a patient's admission and treatment plan. In addition, they provide background information and history not only on the current hospitalization but also on previous medical and surgical events, treatments, social and family history, allergies, and current medications as well as other essential elements of the patient's current condition.

Timely and accurate healthcare documentation facilitates continuity of care for the patient so that all caregivers have the same information to aid them in making the best healthcare decisions quickly and decisively. Delays in treatment and potential patient safety risks increase significantly when reports do not arrive in a timely manner or when they contain errors or omissions.

While most facilities develop their own policies around turnaround times, some acute care TAT requirements have been established by The Joint Commission and are noted below.

- *Consultation*: No standard or requirement time is currently outlined. However, most facilities adopt a 24-hour-or-less TAT policy for consultation reports, as continuity of care and decisions for ongoing treatment may be based on this information.
- *Discharge summary*: The Joint Commission does not outline TAT requirements for discharge summaries.
- *History and physical examination*: The Joint Commission outlines that this report must be in the patient's chart within 24 hours of admission.
- *Operative reports and high-risk procedures*: The Joint Commission outlines that operative reports and other high-risk procedures must have a history and physical examination recorded in the patient's chart before any surgery or procedure can be performed.

Additionally, reports must be dictated or written immediately after an operative or other high-risk procedure; they are to be authenticated by the licensed independent practitioner, and they are to be made available in the medical record as soon as possible after the procedure.

CRITICAL THINKING EXERCISE 9-2

A young man with weakness and lethargy visits an outpatient clinic. He tells the family nurse practitioner (FNP) that he feels like he has a bad case of the flu. He states he has had drenching night sweats and has lost 10 pounds since becoming ill. He is anxious and admits that he has had unprotected sex with two male partners over the past few months. The FNP examines the patient, documenting fever and swollen lymph nodes in his neck. Given this history, what disorder might this young man have? What tests would confirm it? To what specialty would the FNP refer the patient for treatment?

Formatting Acute Care Reports

Demographics

The demographics area of a patient's record includes information about the patient that is not primarily medical in nature. It is contact information for the patient and other identifiers unique to the patient. Patient demographics can consist of details such as those found in Table 9-1.

Some demographics, such as the date of service or patient's medical record number, are manually entered by the dictator by way of a technology interface, but other facts are dictated by the physician for input by the healthcare documentation specialist (HDS). With most modern dictation platforms, the demographic information is captured automatically by the system at the point of dictation and is electronically associated with the transcribed record. HDSs who are editing via modern dictation platforms are often required to verify that the dictated text and the patient information match to ensure accurate demographic mapping. In settings where this is not automated, the HDS may have to manually access the information to verify the patient's demographics. For example, there could be many patients with the name Jonathan Jones. It is the duty of the HDS to use identifiers dictated to determine the correct Jonathan Jones. If minimal information is provided and the correct patient cannot be identified or matched to the record, the HDS should flag the report and notify a supervisor, manager, or quality assurance specialist, per the facility's protocol.

Consultation Report (Consult)

As noted in Chapter 7, consultation reports are sometimes formatted as a letter. Consultations include an examination, review, and assessment of a patient by a healthcare provider other than the attending physician. The letter containing the consultant's findings is usually directed to the requesting physician or attending physician. It may contain personal information if the requesting physician or attending physician and the consultant are friends; for example, first names may be used in the salutation and closing. The following are headings frequently included in a consultation report:

HISTORY AND PHYSICAL EXAMINATION

DIAGNOSTIC STUDIES

ASSESSMENT, DIAGNOSIS, or DIFFERENTIAL DIAGNOSIS

RECOMMENDATION or PLAN

🧠 A&P BRAIN DRAIN BOX 9-3

Groupings of lymph nodes can be found where in the body?

Discharge Summary

The discharge summary (DS) outlines the course of the patient's stay during hospitalization, including reason for hospitalization, significant findings, treatment, any procedures performed, condition of the patient upon discharge, and recommended treatment upon discharge. The following are headings commonly included in a DS:

ADMITTING DIAGNOSIS

DISCHARGE DIAGNOSIS

CHIEF COMPLAINT

HISTORY OF PRESENT ILLNESS

HOSPITAL COURSE

PROGNOSIS

PLAN, DISCHARGE PLAN, or DISPOSITION

DISCHARGE INSTRUCTIONS

CONDITION

TABLE 9-1 PATIENT DEMOGRAPHICS CATEGORIES

Name	Address	Phone Number
Date of Birth	Gender	Race/Ethnicity
Preferred Language	Religion	Insurance Information
Emergency Contact Person	Occupation	Social Security Number
Medical Record Number	Date of Visit	Date of Procedure
Date of Service	Date of Surgery	Date of Examination
Primary Care Physician	Consulting Physician	Surgeon

Emergency Department Report

The emergency department (ED) report is dictated as quickly as possible after care has been rendered, especially if the patient's condition is critical. It is important that subsequent care providers have access to the patient's history, studies obtained, and treatment rendered while the patient was in the ED on which to make decisions and base subsequent care and progress of the patient. Although headings included within an ED report vary among facilities, the following are commonly found:

CHIEF COMPLAINT
HISTORY OF PRESENT ILLNESS
REVIEW OF SYSTEMS
PAST MEDICAL HISTORY
PAST SURGICAL HISTORY
ALLERGIES
CURRENT MEDICATIONS
PHYSICAL EXAMINATION
LABORATORY/DIAGNOSTIC STUDIES
EMERGENCY DEPARTMENT COURSE
DIAGNOSIS
DISPOSITION
CONDITION
PLAN or DISCHARGE INSTRUCTIONS

History and Physical Examination

The history and physical examination (H&P), arguably, is one of the most important reports to be included in patient records. It is a detailed summary of the patient's reason for presentation. Although headings included within an H&P vary among facilities, the following are commonly found:

CHIEF COMPLAINT
HISTORY OF PRESENT ILLNESS
PAST MEDICAL HISTORY
ALLERGIES
CURRENT MEDICATIONS
REVIEW OF SYSTEMS
PHYSICAL EXAMINATION
MENTAL STATUS EXAMINATION
DIAGNOSTIC STUDIES
DIAGNOSIS
ORDERS

Operative Report

The operative report is a summary that details a surgical procedure in chronologic order. Common headings for operative reports include:

PREOPERATIVE DIAGNOSIS
POSTOPERATIVE DIAGNOSIS
REASON FOR OPERATION or INDICATIONS
SURGEON
ASSISTANTS
ANESTHESIOLOGIST
ANESTHESIA
INDICATIONS FOR PROCEDURE
FINDINGS
PROCEDURE, OPERATIVE COURSE, or TECHNIQUE
COMPLICATIONS
TOURNIQUET TIME
HARDWARE
DRAINS
SPECIMENS
ESTIMATED BLOOD LOSS
INSTRUMENT, SPONGE, AND NEEDLE COUNTS
DISPOSITION OF PATIENT
FOLLOWUP

With any area of the record that is highly repetitive in nature, physicians often use "normals," or customized templates of text in the electronic health record. The HDS should pay close attention to areas in which normals are used and edit appropriately. The dictation may be to "use normal template A," for example, with the information in the template unchanged. The dictation may be to "use normal template B" with some parts of the template updated. It is the HDS's responsibility to double check these templates, making sure they fit with the patient on whom they are being dictated for gender, age, and disease process.

Keep in mind that acute care reports being formatted and viewed in an electronic environment do not require page breaks or subsequent page headers because formatting is automatically generated by the technology. Follow facility guidelines to allow text to wrap from the beginning of the report to the end without adding page breaks.

Acute care reports that are formatted outside of an electronic environment or that will be printed should contain continuation information. For each subsequent page, "(Continued)" must be entered at the end of the page. The header at the top of the following page should contain the patient's name, medical record number (where applicable), the date of service or the date of procedure/operation, and the page number. Additional identifying information may be included in the header according to facility preference. Subsequent pages must contain at least two lines of text from the body of the report. Do not leave a signature line or a sign-off block alone on a page.

CRITICAL THINKING EXERCISE 9-3

The laboratory data in a report you are editing include a urinalysis. As part of that result, the dictation is, "Specific gravity greater than ten thirty-five." What is the normal range for specific gravity? What exactly do you transcribe and why?

Model Report 3 in this chapter shows how a report that includes continuation information should appear. All other reports within this text are shown without page breaks or continuation information.

N.B.: The list of reports, headings, and formatting instructions included for acute care reports is not all inclusive but is intended to give the student HDS or medical editor a broad overall view of the acute care hospital setting for patients and patient medical records. Refer to Appendix G for more resources.

A&P BRAIN DRAIN BOX 9-4

Which blood vessels contain valves?

INDEX OF ACUTE CARE REPORTS

Student Name: _____   Date: _____

ID Number	Patient Name	Type of Report/Procedure
S-9	David Robert Lepinski	Oromaxillofacial surgery
S-11	Dinah Cash	Obstetrics/gynecology surgery
S-14	Adam Ward	Oromaxillofacial surgery
S-17	Simone Dahl	Orthopedic surgery
S-19	Melvin Arney	Ear, nose, and throat surgery
S-23	Deborah Keith	Plastic surgery report
S-31	Ursula Castro	Plastic surgery report
S-32	Thomas A. Clegg	General surgery report
S-33	Beldon Kays	Genitourinary surgery report
S-34	Jerry Graham	Orthopedic surgery report
S-38	Ladonna Young	Obstetrics/gynecology surgery
S-43	Lightbourne Byfield	Orthopedic surgery report
S-46	Tina Jane Wolfe	Orthopedic surgical report
S-47	Anthony L. Duckett	Ear, nose, and throat surgical report
S-49	Lori Anne Richey	General surgery report
S-56	Joe Christopher Lanier	General surgery
S-61	Mary Louise Bright	Obstetrics/gynecology surgery
S-64	Jerry Watson	Vascular surgery
S-65	Trent R. Lockwood	Oromaxillofacial surgery
S-66	Michael R. Turnbow	General surgery
S-70	Leena O. Martin	Vascular surgery
S-71	Leslie S. Hunter	Ear, nose, and throat surgery
S-72	Stephen M. Joyner	Orthopedic surgery
S-75	Laura I. Benson	General surgery
S-81	Jonathan T. Weeks	Genitourinary surgery
S-82	Aimee J. Fitzgerald	Obstetrics/gynecology surgery
S-83	Doris Vanham	Nephrology surgery
S-86	Randall Oscar Doubletree	Genitourinary surgery
S-87	Miguel Cantu	Orthopedic surgery
S-90	Troy Gibbons	Genitourinary surgery
S-91	Roberta L. Grissom	Ear, nose, and throat surgery
S-95	Stefanie Woolsey	Orthopedic surgery
S-96	Daniel T. Clark	Ear, nose, and throat surgery
S-97	Starr Kellogg	Obstetrics/gynecology surgery
S-98	Charles L. Looper	Genitourinary surgery
S-99	Lee Weisenhantz	Orthopedic surgery
M-13	Mark N. Scott	Emergency Department Treatment Record
M-20	Tristan R. Leher	Emergency Department Treatment Record
M-26	Gayle Ann Moss	Emergency Department Treatment Record
M-37	Briggs Jackson	Emergency Department Treatment Record
M-42	Don Q. Fogarty	Emergency Department Treatment Record

M-46	Marian Parry	Emergency Department Treatment Record
M-57	Ahmed Saleh	Emergency Department Treatment Record
M-66	John Doe	Emergency Department Treatment Record
M-69	James E. Stevenson	Emergency Department Treatment Record
M-84	Steve Fowler	Emergency Department Treatment Record
M-87	Paul Travis Overton	Emergency Department Treatment Record
M-90	Michael John Babjak	Emergency Department Treatment Record
M-93	Salvatore Menchaca	Emergency Department Treatment Record
M-96	Leonard Gonzales	Emergency Department Treatment Record

CHAPTER 10

CHRONIC CARE

LEARNING OBJECTIVES

1. Discuss the differences between a clinician and a surgeon.
2. Discuss the circumstances under which a surgeon would require a patient consultation.
3. Give four benefits of electronic healthcare records.
4. List how Progress Reports are formatted.
5. Name the advantages of an HDS working in chronic care. Are there any disadvantages?

INTRODUCTION

The chronic care of patients consists of medical care given in physician offices and clinics in an outpatient setting. It is given by doctors, physician assistants, nurses or nurse practitioners, physical therapists, occupational therapists, mental health therapists, massage therapists, acupuncturists, dentists or dental hygienists, and others who deliver medical care. Chronic care can be received anywhere and everywhere patients are seen other than in an acute care setting, including in the home.

Chronic care patients have one or more preexisting or long-term medical ailments that require ongoing treatment and checkups by the primary care physician and other specialists who consult or participate in the patient's care. In private practices, many physicians have implemented electronic medical records (EMR) systems. These EMRs may or may not be linked to bigger electronic healthcare records (EHR) systems through interoperability. Until interoperability is able to be implemented nationwide, in which multiple healthcare providers and facilities would have full access to all of a patient's medical records, there will continue to be challenges in having the full picture regarding a patient's past history, current diseases or disorders, and treatment.

Using these information systems, individual patient care is tracked to manage chronic illness or provide preventive care. The entire healthcare team uses the information within the EMR and EHR to guide the course of treatment, anticipate problems, and track progress. Overall, the ability to share information (keeping HIPAA laws inviolate) has led to the faster and safer delivery of patient care.

Outpatient reports dictated in a clinical setting include:

Followup Notes

History, Physical, Impression, Plan (HPIP) notes

Subjective, Objective, Assessment, Plan (SOAP) notes

Progress Notes

History and Physical Examinations

Consultations

Discharge Summaries

The following model reports are examples of the types of reports seen in the chronic care setting. See "Formatting Chronic Care Reports" on page 95 for more details.

🧠 A&P BRAIN DRAIN BOX 10-1

List the three cycles of human hair.

MODEL REPORT 1: CHRONIC CARE

VASCULAR/NEUROVASCULAR SURGERY FOLLOWUP NOTE

Patient Name: James E. Stotler   **PCP**: Chris Salem, DO
Date of Exam: 08/03/----   **Age/Sex**: 79/M
ID#: M-17

CHIEF COMPLAINT: Bilateral lower extremity pain with ambulation.

HISTORY: The patient is a 79-year-old Caucasian gentleman who is currently being evaluated for a diarrheal illness for the last year. He states that over the last several years his walking has become incrementally worse based upon pain in his calves with walking. Started mostly on the left but does involve both relatively equally. The pain is consistent at about 5 to 6 blocks currently. When it initially started, it was mostly at longer distances. He does state that if he pushes it, it starts to move up into his thighs. If he really, really "goes after it," the pain may come up into his buttocks. He denies postprandial pain. Denies TIAs or stroke-like symptoms. His cardiovascular risk factors include coronary artery disease. He has hypertension and hyperlipidemia, for which he is medically controlled. He denies having diabetes, and he quit smoking in 1998 after a 40-pack-year history. He does have a history of mild congestive heart failure, although he has never had a heart attack. He denies having any active chest, left shoulder, or jaw pain.

MEDICATIONS: Currently include niacin, metoprolol, lisinopril, cilostazol, simvastatin, and pantoprazole.

ALLERGIES: No known drug allergies.

PHYSICAL EXAMINATION: VITAL SIGNS: Temperature 97, left arm pressure is 113/56, right arm pressure is 109/80, pulse is 88, respirations 19. He has easily palpable normal upper extremity pulses with easily palpable subclavian arteries bilaterally. No supraclavicular bruits. He has 2+ carotid pulses bilaterally with good upstroke and bilateral bruits. He has easily palpable superficial temporal pulses. He has no epigastric pulsation, no epigastric or flank bruits. He has diminished femoral pulses bilaterally, but they are palpable, and he has had no palpable pulses below this bilaterally. He has stigmata of peripheral vascular disease at his distal leg and foot level; however, he has no tissue breakdown.

DIAGNOSTIC DATA: Imaging and noninvasive vascular laboratory data: He underwent lower extremity segmental pressures and PVRs on July 19 of this year, which revealed evidence of multilevel occlusive disease bilaterally. This is moderate to severe in nature with a right ABI of 0.5 and a left ABI of 0.7. On the left it does appear the majority of his disease is actually in the SFA/popliteal region, and his right-sided disease is multifactorial with both aortoiliac and superficial femoral popliteal disease. His toe pressure on the right is 49. His toe pressure on the left is 44. His PVRs do reveal a bit of blunting and some latency, suggesting multilevel disease bilaterally.

(Continued)

Patient Name: James E. Stotler
Date of Exam: 08/03/----
ID#: M-17
Page 2

IMPRESSION/PLAN: Overall, Mr. Stotler states that this is not greatly limiting him. I discussed with him a structured walking program and that he should again start to walk. There is no danger with this.

After claudication education and a discussion of intermittent claudication, I discussed with him that he needs, as well, an aortic screening and a carotid duplex. Based upon his segmental pressures, we will see him again in 6 months with an aortoiliac duplex and ABIs to evaluate for progression.

He understands this and will begin his structured walking program. I believe that, from a medical standpoint, he appears to be overall well controlled. He is on a beta blocker, an ACE inhibitor, and a statin medication. Further, he is already taking 100 mg b.i.d. of cilostazol. I gave him my card and said that he can follow up with us sooner if need be.

_____

Ly An Tabor, MD, Vascular Surgery

LAT:xx
D: 08/04/----
T: 08/04/----

c: Chris Salem, DO, Family Practice

MODEL REPORT 2

BONE MARROW TRANSPLANT CLINIC FOLLOWUP NOTE

Patient Name: Rodolfo Garcia   **PCP**: Solomon T. Fisher, MD
Date of Exam: 7/1/----   **Age/Sex**: 25/M
ID#: M-28

INTRODUCTION: Rodolfo Garcia is a 25-year-old Hispanic male, day +4 status post a reduced-intensity, matched, related transplant for non-Hodgkin lymphoma, who is seen today in followup.

HISTORY: Patient is doing well overall. He denies nausea, vomiting, diarrhea, and rash. He is eating and drinking well.

REVIEW OF SYSTEMS: Patient denies fevers, sore throat, mucositis, shortness of breath, chest pain, abdominal pain, dysuria, hematuria, hematochezia, epistaxis, and chills.

MEDICATIONS
1. Coumadin 8 mg daily.
2. AcipHex 20 mg daily p.r.n.
3. Fluconazole 400 mg daily.
4. Acyclovir 800 mg b.i.d.
5. Magnesium 400 mg b.i.d.
6. Tacrolimus 2 mg b.i.d.
7. Actigall 600 mg a.m. and 300 mg p.m.
8. Levaquin 500 mg daily.

PHYSICAL EXAMINATION: Temperature 96.9, blood pressure 119/80, pulse 85, respirations 20, weight 67.1 kg, oxygen saturation 98% on room air. GENERAL: No acute distress. HEENT: Sclerae nonicteric. Sinuses are nontender. Oral mucosa is clear. Lungs are clear to auscultation bilaterally. HEART: Regular rate and rhythm without murmurs, rubs, or gallops. Extremities are without edema. Skin is without rash. PICC line is without erythema, tenderness, or discharge.

LABORATORY DATA: White blood cells 0.7, hemoglobin 13.2, platelets 92,000. Creatinine 0.8, magnesium 1.2, potassium 4.5.

IMPRESSION: This is a 25-year-old male, day +4 post a reduced-intensity, matched, related transplant. Overall he is doing well.

PLAN: Patient will follow up with me in clinic tomorrow. Will stop Coumadin when platelet count is greater than 80,000.

_____

Solomon T. Fisher, MD, Hematology

STF:xx
D: 7/1/----
T: 7/2/----

MODEL REPORT 3

PHYSICAL MEDICINE AND REHABILITATION CONSULTATION

Patient Name: Valerie Smith   **PCP**: Susan McGinness
Date of Consultation: 03/10/----   **Age/Sex**: 59/F
ID#: M-2

REASON FOR CONSULTATION: Recurrent back pain with intermittent right sciatica.

HISTORY OF PRESENT ILLNESS: Ms. Smith is a 59-year-old female who presents to me with an acute exacerbation of her chronic intermittent back pain with some associated right radicular/neurogenic leg pain. The patient states that initially she had a severe back pain episode in 1993. Then her first combined back pain with sciatica occurred in 1996. She subsequently underwent a myelogram, which demonstrated combined congenital and acquired spinal stenosis at L4-5 and less so at L5-S1. Eventually her sciatica pain improved, but she has had recurrent bouts of back pain, slightly worse on the right, over subsequent years. She had a recent exacerbation at the beginning of this week in which she awakened with no precipitating injury, activity, or other known variable. She presents today indicating that her back pain represents 100% of her pain while sitting; but while standing and walking, the back pain represents only about 70% of her total pain, with the right lateral thigh pain and occasionally slightly further than her knee representing the other 30% of her pain. Her pain is generally aggravated with any type of activity, particularly stooping, bending, and lifting, as well as with prolonged standing and walking. The pain is a combination of a dull ache across her back and a slightly sharper shooting pain down the right leg. Her pain severity now ranges from a 4/10 to a 9/10.

NEUROLOGIC REVIEW OF SYSTEMS: Remarkable for the intermittent right sciatica in a predominantly L5 distribution. She will have some associated numbness and paresthesias on the right lateral ankle and foot, dorsal region, in a partial L5 dermatomal distribution. She occasionally feels some weakness in the right leg, particularly when the sciatica pain has worsened. Denies bowel or bladder changes or incontinence.

CONSTITUTIONAL REVIEW OF SYSTEMS: Unremarkable for fevers, chills, night sweats, malaise, weight loss, history of malignancy, or recent infection. Treatment for this back pain has consisted only of some analgesic medications. Patient has had no recent physical therapy and has had no injections for this back problem. Furthermore, she is unable to do any specific exercises at this time, although she does attempt some low-impact cardiovascular conditioning when the pain is not exacerbated.

PAST HISTORY: Probable viral myocarditis with secondary residual cardiomyopathy (ejection fraction ranging from 35% to 45%), associated intermittent ventricular tachycardia, and hyperlipidemia.

(Continued)

Patient Name: Valerie Smith
Date of Consultation: 03/10/----
ID#: M-2
Page 2

PAST SURGICAL HISTORY: Noncontributory.

SOCIAL HISTORY: Denies tobacco use and alcohol use. Her current job is that of a linguist with the Defense Language Institute.

MEDICATIONS: Current analgesics consist of Skelaxin 800 mg 1 tablet p.o. t.i.d. p.r.n., tramadol 1 to 2 tablets q.i.d. p.r.n. (generally uses only one of these tablets daily). Other meds include Coreg, ramipril, Zocor, and Aleve.

PHYSICAL EXAMINATION

GENERAL APPEARANCE: Well-nourished, well-developed female in mild distress, alert and oriented x4, pleasant, cooperative, and appropriate.

Spine
- Posture/Inspection: Obvious list/shift to the right while sitting, particularly more evident while standing.
- Lumbopelvic AROM: Patient has aggravation of the lumbosacral-area back pain with flexion greater than 60 degrees, even more so with extension, particularly on the right side, in which she has exacerbation of the right lumbosacral area with greater than 10 degrees.
- Palpation: Tenderness is noted over the lumbosacral region.

Neurologic
- Gait: Able to do heel-toe and tandem walking for a few steps.
- Motor: There is 5/5 in all muscle groups in the lower extremities.
- Sensory: Diminished light touch and pinprick is evident on the right lateral ankle and foot, dorsum, in a partial L5 dermatome; the remaining portions of the lower extremities arc intact to light touch and pinprick.
- Reflexes: Patella is 2+ and symmetric. Achilles 2- and symmetric with a normal flexion response to Babinski testing.
- Nerve tension signs: Positive reproduction of some of the right buttock and lateral leg thigh pain with a right straight-leg raise; however, this does not go beyond that of the popliteal fossa. The left side is unremarkable.

Extremities/Vascular
Normal temperature and coloration of the distal legs and feet with palpable dorsalis pedis pulses and without cyanosis or edema.

X-RAY DATA: CT myelogram done in the late 1980s demonstrated some combined degenerative and congenital L4-5 greater than L5-S1 canal stenosis with some disk protrusions at L4-5 greater than L5-S1 and facet arthropathy.

(Continued)

Patient Name: Valerie Smith
Date of Consultation: 03/10/----
ID#: M-2
Page 3

ASSESSMENT: Recurrent right L4-5 greater than L5-S1 herniated nucleus pulposus (HNP), protrusion type, with associated canal stenosis and secondary mechanical low back pain as well as intermittent right L5 neurogenic leg claudication.

PLAN
1. Naprosyn 500 mg 1 tablet b.i.d.
2. Vicodin 1 to 2 tablets q.i.d. p.r.n. increased pain along with the Skelaxin p.r.n. difficulty with sleep.
3. Will obtain x-rays of her lumbosacral spine today.
4. Lumbosacral magnetic resonance imaging scan (MRI) to better assess the soft tissue, disk, and neural structures as well as the severity of the canal stenosis.
5. Physical therapy for core stabilization,
6. Patient will return to clinic after obtaining the MRI, as well as begin a physical therapy program.

_____
Carlos Bautista, MD
Physical Medicine and Rehabilitation

CB:xx
D: 03/10/----
T: 03/10/----

c: Susan McGinness, MD, Family Practice

MODEL REPORT 4

VASCULAR CLINIC FOLLOWUP NOTE

Patient Name: Benjamin Dunham   **PCP**: Marie Aaron, DO
Date of Exam: 29 Mar ----   **Age/Sex**: 58-year-old male
ID#: M-62

HISTORY: Mr. Dunham is a 58-year-old black man with a history of carotid artery stenosis, status post bilateral CEAs, in 2001 on the left and in 2003 on the right, both of which were widely patent as of 8 Dec ---- when he had his last duplex. Patient also has a history of peripheral vascular disease. Latest imaging done 8 Dec ---- showed a hemodynamically significant superficial femoral artery and bilateral tibial calcification and claudication. The patient has been working on an exercise regime. He has no medications for his peripheral vascular disease and states that his tolerance to exercise is increasing. He walks 1 mile a day, 4 to 5 days a week, walking further and faster before the claudication sets in than previously. He now can walk 400 to 500 yards briskly before the claudication sets in, and he then can walk 1+ mile using a normal gait.

PAST MEDICAL HISTORY: Significant for increased cholesterol and hypertension.

PAST SURGICAL HISTORY: Has had a hernia repair, Lasik surgery, and a vasectomy.

MEDICATIONS: Zocor.

SOCIAL HISTORY: Does not smoke, has not smoked for 8 years, but he had a 30-pack-year history before he quit. He drinks 2 to 6 beers per day.

PHYSICAL EXAMINATION: VITALS show blood pressure to be 78/43 on the left, 95/48 on the right, pulse 84, respirations 17. He is awake, alert, and oriented. LUNGS: Clear to auscultation bilaterally. CARDIOVASCULAR EXAM: S1, S2. Good peripheral pulses. Palpable pulses in the lower extremities. He has good capillary refill. NEUROLOGIC: No focal deficits. Mood is bright.

ASSESSMENT
1. A 58-year-old black male with carotid artery disease, status post bilateral carotid endarterectomies.
2. Peripheral vascular disease, which is improving with exercise.

PLAN: We encouraged Mr. Dunham to continue his exercise and diet regime. We will see him again in approximately 1 month.

_____

Ly An Tabor, MD, Vascular Surgery

LAT:xx
D: 03/29/----
T: 03/30/----

c: Marie Aaron, DO, Family Practice

MODEL REPORT 5

RADIATION ONCOLOGY CLINIC FOLLOWUP NOTE

Patient Name: James L. Matthews   **PCP**: A. Leigh Wells, MD
Date of Exam: 14 June ----   **Age/Sex**: 67-year-old male
ID#: M-72

DIAGNOSES
1. Pathologic T1 versus T2N2b squamous cell carcinoma of the right lateral oral tongue treated with surgery and postoperative radiotherapy 20 years ago.
2. Squamous cell carcinoma of the posterior pharyngeal wall, pathologic stage T2N0, treated with total laryngopharyngectomy and left neck dissection with free flap reconstruction.

The patient received postoperative radiotherapy to the retropharyngeal lymph nodes to a total dose of 57.6 Gy delivered in 1.8 Gy/fraction, completed on 14 March this year due to the finding of suspicious retropharyngeal lymph nodes on the patient's preoperative MRI scan.

HISTORY: The patient returns today in routine followup. A PET CT obtained on 7 June revealed no suspicious FDG uptake. There was a sclerotic lesion in the right pubic ramus, which was thought to be atypical for metastatic disease. Patient's blood work on 9 May indicated a TSH of 7.59 and a free thyroxine of 0.8.

Currently the patient notes persistent ear drainage, which has been quite troublesome. He is using boric acid drops at this time, and he has bilateral myringotomy tubes in place. Otherwise, he notes mild difficulty swallowing either large pieces of food or very dry food. Nevertheless, he has gained 4 pounds over the past 2 months. He notes moderate xerostomia, which does respond to pilocarpine 5 mg in the morning. His taste is 79% recovered. He denies significant pain in the head and neck region.

PHYSICAL EXAMINATION: In general, this is a pleasant, well-appearing Caucasian male in no acute distress. HEENT: Bilateral ear tubes present with drainage noted. Anicteric sclerae. Pupils are equal, round, and reactive to light and accommodation. Extraocular movements intact. Visual inspection of the oral cavity and oropharynx reveals no suspicious mucosal lesions. The mucosa is somewhat dry. NECK: There is a fullness in the left neck compatible with a free flap placement. No palpable adenopathy. The tracheal stoma is intact with no suspicious changes.

IMPRESSION/PLAN: Mr. Matthews is radiographically and clinically without evidence of recurrent head and neck cancer 3 months after having completed a course of re-irradiation to the retropharyngeal lymph nodes for a second head and neck primary. He does have evidence of biochemical hypothyroidism, and he does report heat intolerance; therefore, I have started him on Synthroid 25 mcg daily.

(Continued)

Patient Name: James L. Matthews
Date of Exam: 14 June ----
ID#: M-72
Page 2

He is to follow up with his primary care provider tomorrow, and I have asked patient to notify his PCP of this new diagnosis. Either his PCP or I can follow the patient with serial TSH checks to ensure that the patient is on the appropriate dose of Synthroid.

Otherwise, the patient continues to do well. He is followed closely by the ENT clinic with regular fiberoptic endoscopy, then clinical exams. I will see the patient again in 2 months. In the interval, he will be seen by Dr. David Cohen of Hematology to follow his iron-deficiency anemia.

_____
L. (Lonnie) Willem Erwin, MD
Radiation Oncology

LWE:xx
D: 06/14/----
T: 06/15/----

c: A. Leigh Wells, MD, Internal Medicine
   David H. Cohen, MD, Hematology
   Leah Pittfield, MD, ENT Clinic

MODEL REPORT 6

HEMATOLOGY HISTORY, PHYSICAL, IMPRESSION, PLAN (HPIP NOTE)

Patient Name: Mercedes Daniels   **PCP**: A. Leigh Wells, MD
Date of Exam: 10/22/----   **Sex/Age**: F/39
ID#: M-209

HISTORY: The patient returns in scheduled followup. She received 2 doses of IVIg, one on September 17 and the second on October 15. Platelets on September 17 had been down to 20,000, and they were bumped up to 124,000. On October 15 platelets were down to 41,000 and are now 115,000. Her only complaint is that of her heart "pounding" at night. She does not notice this during the day, but when she lies down and wears her oxygen, she seems to notice it more. No other new complaints. Right elbow continues to hurt, but this is not terrible pain and is not worrisome.

PHYSICAL EXAM: VITAL SIGNS: BP 121/73, P 85, R 20, T 96.7, weight 128 pounds. CONSTITUTIONAL: Well-developed, well-nourished, healthy-appearing, young white female with obvious Down syndrome in no acute distress. HENT and NECK: Normocephalic, atraumatic. Facies typical for Down syndrome. Oropharynx without mucosal lesions, no breakdown of oral mucosa. No palpable petechiae. Geographic tongue. Mucous membranes are beefy red. No thrush noted, and this is stable for her. Edentulous. Nares normal. TMs not examined. Neck is shortened without masses or JVD. Thyroid with no enlargement, tenderness, or masses. EYES: PERRLA/EOMI. Sclerae anicteric. Conjunctivae, lids normal. Funduscopic exam not done. CHEST: Respiratory effort normal. Scattered expiratory wheezes at times, fairly clear otherwise. CARDIOVASCULAR: PMI is markedly displaced at the lateral margin of the chest cavity. Diastolic and systolic murmurs heard with varying crescendo-decrescendo qualities, grade 2/6 for both. Continuous murmur goes through S1 and S2 with a possible S3 gallop. No rubs. Carotid, femoral, and pedal pulses normal but symmetrically diminished. BREASTS: Not reexamined. ABDOMEN: Body habitus consistent with truncal obesity. Normal bowel sounds. Soft, nontender, protuberant with no hepatosplenomegaly or masses, no rebound or guarding. GU, PELVIC, and RECTAL deferred. LYMPHATIC: No abnormal lymph nodes in cervical, axillary, or groin areas. MUSCULOSKELETAL: Exam of bones, joints, muscles of extremities, neck, spine, ribs, and pelvis for gait, range of motion, and function appears normal. EXTREMITIES: Typical features of Down syndrome with short hands, no webbing. No cyanosis, clubbing, clots, or edema. SKIN: Discoloration of the nail beds, which are more cyanotic than previously. Mild perioral cyanosis as well. Petechial rash on both feet extending to her midshins, improved. Apparent deposition of old hemosiderin, no evidence of worsening, currently less red than when her platelets were very low. Large, healed skin defect on the anterior surface of her left hand that looks like a healed burn. NEUROLOGIC: Cranial nerves grossly intact, nonfocal. Sensation, strength, and mental status are normal for her. PSYCHIATRIC: Mood, affect are normal for her.

LAB values show CBC with platelets 115,000, Hgb 14.6, Hct 44.3, WBC 3.1. Chem panel is within normal limits.

(Continued)

IMPRESSION

1. The patient is a 39-year-old white female with Down syndrome who was diagnosed with probable medication-induced versus immune-based thrombocytopenia. She was treated with steroids with improvement. Her platelet count returned to near normal, and steroids were thus tapered. This recurred, and I think it is most consistent with idiopathic thrombocytopenic purpura (ITP). Because of the fear of chronic steroids in this particular patient with her volume overload, congestive heart failure, and essentially poor underlying cardiac reserve, she has received IVIg approximately every four weeks with a nice bump in her platelets to greater than 100,000. I have tried to back off on that, but she requires it about q.4 weeks; therefore, I will plan to keep her on it. She has petechiae as a manifestation of disease but has suffered no overt, large bleeds. Despite taking a long time to receive the IVIg, she tolerates it very well, better than I think she would tolerate chronic steroids. The other option, of course, would be splenectomy; however, with her compromised cardiac picture, I am hesitant to have that done.

2. Congestive heart failure with atherosclerotic disease and multiple valvular abnormalities, initially considered for surgical intervention; however, this is not likely to happen since she is currently beyond her life expectancy with her diagnosis. Her mother wants to do nothing to hasten her death. On today's exam she had some decompensation with worsened peripheral and persistent perioral cyanosis. I think her heart disease is worsening. Patient continues to use O2 at night, and I have asked her mother to elevate the head of her daughter's bed. This may help her sensation of a pounding heart.

3. Right upper extremity pain, unclear etiology, an intermittent complaint.

4. Previous mild abdominal pain, likely menstrual, resolved.

PLAN

1. CBC every week.
2. IVIg every four weeks.
3. Return in eight weeks with CBC and CMP prior.

_____

David H. Cohen, MD, Hematology

DHC:xx
D: 10/22/----
T: 10/25/----

MODEL REPORT 7

INFECTIOUS DISEASE
SUBJECTIVE, OBJECTIVE, ASSESSMENT, PLAN (SOAP NOTE)

Patient Name: Jimmy McGann   **PCP**: Beth Brian, MD
Date of Exam: 12/29/----   **Sex/Age**: M/35
ID#: M-210

CHIEF COMPLAINT: Nonproductive cough with congestion.

SUBJECTIVE: This patient with a history of AIDS, status post Pneumocystis carinii pneumonia, herpes esophagitis, perirectal herpes, and CMV hepatitis, is seen today for the first time in 4-1/2 months. The patient indicates that in mid-November he stopped all his medications because, "I just got confused about the dosing." When I asked why he had not called, he said he just never thought about it. He relates that his most acute problem right now is the development of a nonproductive cough associated with congestion. There have been no fevers, chills, pleuritic chest pain, anorexia, nausea, vomiting, increased diarrhea, or GU symptoms.

OBJECTIVE: HEENT are basically unrevealing with no posterior drainage. Neck supple, good range of motion, no significant adenopathy. Back exam benign. Chest is relatively clear, although he does have diminished breath sounds in the bases. Cardiovascular: S1, S2 without rubs or murmurs. Abdomen: Bowel sounds present. Abdomen is soft, nontender with no guarding or rebound. Extremities are unrevealing. Skin clear. No rashes, ulcerations, or lesions at this time.

ASSESSMENT
1. Bronchitis. At this point, I think the prudent thing is to address this problem acutely with Zithromax and Tussionex.
2. History of acquired immunodeficiency syndrome. Once again, I reviewed how critical it is for him to maintain compliance and followup. I have expressed that if I am going to make a 100% commitment to him, he likewise has to commit to his own health care. As such, if he fails to return in followup, we will have to seek an alternative physician to provide his care. He indicates that he understands my concern and anxiety. I have stated that we are going to deal with his acute illness, and then I will place him back on his medications. Repeat labs today to assess his status.
3. Cytomegalovirus hepatitis. We will recheck his liver functions.
4. Status post herpes of esophagus and perirectal area. No current symptoms.

(Continued)

Patient Name: Jimmy McGann
Date of Exam: 12/29/----
ID#: M-210
Page 2

PLAN
1. Z-Pak.
2. Tussionex 5 mL q.12 h. p.r.n.
3. CBC, Chem-18, CD4 count, and viral load.
4. Return in 10 to 14 days to review data and make some decisions about his future therapy.

_____

Beth Brian, MD, Infectious Disease

BB:xx
D: 12/29/----
T: 12/30/----

CRITICAL THINKING EXERCISE 10-1

While teaching a healthcare documentation specialist class, one of the students asks if it is ever okay to transcribe without using a headset; for example, using their speakers. How should the instructor reply?

STYLES AND STANDARDS

Some types of reports used in chronic care are formatted similarly to acute care reports; others, such as a Progress Note or SOAP Note, are more brief forms of placing status updates in the record and may be less structured than acute care reports. The terms "chronic care" and "clinical care" for the purposes of this text refer to other than surgical or acute care.

Surgeons versus Clinicians: These titles are used according to the disciplines in which each specializes. All doctors are teachers; they learn a philosophy in medical school of "see one, do one, teach one." Doctors often will teach at a local medical school while keeping office hours in addition to being on staff at one or more hospitals. A surgeon is a physician who treats disease, injury, and deformity by operation or a manipulation procedure. Surgeons hold office hours and see patients in a clinical setting where examinations are performed with preoperative testing done according to each patient's need. Clinicians, on the other hand, specialize in the nonsurgical approach to medicine. The clinician is in charge of the day-to-day care of patients and their ongoing health needs. If and when surgery becomes a part of that health need, the clinician will call a surgeon in consultation. Together they work toward the patient's full recovery, including any and all ancillary healthcare personnel necessary to achieve that goal.

Formatting Chronic Care Reports

Consultation Report (Consult)

As noted in Chapter 7, consultation reports are sometimes formatted as a letter. Consultations include an examination, review, and assessment of a patient by a healthcare provider other than the attending physician. The letter, containing the consultant's findings, is usually directed to the requesting physician/attending physician. It may contain personal information if the requesting physician/attending physician and the

consultant are friends; for example, first names may be used in the salutation and closing. The following are headings included in a consultation report:

HISTORY AND PHYSICAL EXAMINATION
DIAGNOSTIC STUDIES
ASSESSMENT, DIAGNOSIS, or DIFFERENTIAL DIAGNOSIS
RECOMMENDATION or PLAN

History, Physical, Impression, Plan (HPIP) notes

HPIP notes are similar in nature to a progress note and the format of a SOAP note, a well-recognized type of followup note. However, the HPIP include the headings: history, physical, impression, and plan. These headings are self-explanatory in that a brief, pertinent patient history is included under the History heading, the physical examination is catalogued under Physical, the diagnosis is listed under Impression, and the plan for further care and treatment is outlined under Plan.

HISTORY
PHYSICAL
IMPRESSION
PLAN

Subjective, Objective, Assessment, Plan (SOAP) notes

Physicians most often use the acronym SOAP when referring to this type of report. The SOAP note is a type of progress note but with specific headings: subjective, objective, assessment, and plan. Included after the Subjective heading is all information related to history. The physical examination findings are placed under the Objective heading. The patient's diagnosis or diagnoses are listed under Assessment, and the Plan portion of the note contains any "next steps"

 CRITICAL THINKING EXERCISE 10-2

While editing an infectious disease report, a medical editor discovers that her sister's boyfriend has tested HIV-positive. She would like to protect her sister from harm and is considering telling her about her boyfriend's health status. Being a professional in a healthcare-related field, is this okay?

information regarding the patient's care; for example, changes in medication, the addition of physical therapy, consultations that will be obtained, or whether surgery will be required.

SUBJECTIVE

OBJECTIVE

ASSESSMENT

PLAN

History and Physical Examination (H&P)

As noted in Chapter 9, the history and physical examination is an important report to be included in patient records. Whether an initial H&P or a preoperative H&P, it is a detailed summary of the patient's reason for presentation. While headings included within an H&P vary between facilities, the following are commonly found:

CHIEF COMPLAINT

HISTORY OF PRESENT ILLNESS

PAST MEDICAL HISTORY

ALLERGIES

CURRENT MEDICATIONS

REVIEW OF SYSTEMS

PHYSICAL EXAMINATION

MENTAL STATUS EXAMINATION

DIAGNOSTIC STUDIES

DIAGNOSIS

ORDERS

Progress Notes (also called Followup Notes)

Progress notes are dictated by the physician to chronicle ongoing patient care for chronic illness in an outpatient setting. Progress notes may be dictated as simple paragraphs of narrative text or in the SOAP format. Progress notes have no standardized headings or subheadings.

Keep in mind that chronic care reports being formatted and viewed in an electronic environment do not require page breaks or subsequent page headers because formatting is automatically generated by the technology. Follow facility guidelines to allow text to wrap from the beginning of the report to the end without adding page breaks.

Chronic care reports that are formatted outside of an electronic environment or that will be printed should contain continuation information. For each subsequent page, "(Continued)" must be entered at the end of the page. The header at the top of the following page should contain the patient's name, medical record number (where applicable), the date of examination or consultation, and the page number. Additional identifying information may be included in the header according to facility preference. Subsequent pages must contain at least two lines of text from the body of the report. Do not leave a signature line or a sign-off block alone on a page.

Model Report 2 in this chapter shows how a report that includes continuation information should appear. All other reports within this text are shown without page breaks or continuation information.

CRITICAL THINKING EXERCISE 10-3

A medical editor has started a new job; while working, he detects medical errors in a report. He inquires of his team leader how to proceed—for example, should he flag this report for QA? The team leader tells the medical editor that this MTSO does not allow flagging of reports. He feels uncomfortable leaving medical errors, but how should he proceed?

INDEX OF CHRONIC CARE REPORTS

Student Name: _____   Date: _____

ID Number	Patient Name	Type of Report/Procedure
M-1	E. Sinks McClarty	Bone marrow transplant clinic followup
M-3	Natalie Birch	Orthopedic clinic
M-5	Raul Jaramillo	Vascular surgery clinic followup note
M-6	Christopher R. Burke	Preoperative history and physical examination
M-7	Michele Bourn	Colorectal surgery consultation
M-9	Kazuo Matsui	Radiation oncology consultation
M-10	Lance Everett	Bone marrow transplant clinic followup note
M-12	Adam L. Berkman	Vascular surgery clinic followup note
M-15	Joel Flores	Radiation oncology clinic followup note
M-16	Arthur T. Richeson	Vascular surgery followup note
M-18	Richard J. Fisher	Hematology/Oncology bone marrow transplant followup note
M-19	Jack T. Lampe, PhD	Internal medicine clinic note
M-23	Daniel J. Tremblay	Internal medicine followup note
M-24	Otto Rentz	Hematology/Oncology clinic outpatient progress note
M-27	Lisa Marie Jones	Orthopedic clinic consultation
M-31	Leonard C. Thomas	Colorectal surgery consultation
M-34	Jennifer Ann Adcock	Orthopedic surgery followup note
M-36	Kelsi Shaffer	Orthopedic followup note
M-39	Frieda Kasanjian	Vascular surgery followup note
M-41	Sheena Ferruzzi	Colorectal surgery consultation
M-43	Joel Flores	Radiation oncology followup note
M-45	Curtis L. Johnson	Bone marrow followup note
M-47	Robert M. Sager	Orthopedic surgery followup note
M-48	Hamilton Jones	Vascular surgery consultation
M-51	Christopher Lee	Orthopedic clinic consultation
M-54	Juan Gutierrez	Oromaxillofacial surgery consultation
M-55	Melissa Baker	Discharge summary
M-56	Jerry Graham	Preop history and physical examination
M-60	Tashinda Jones	Plastic surgery clinic followup note
M-61	Eduardo Martinez	Nephrology clinic followup note
M-63	Jennifer Santinos	Neurology/Orthopedics discharge summary
M-65	Hilda Schmidt	Radiation Oncology clinic note
M-67	Fergus Roberts	Vascular surgery clinic consultation
M-68	Brian Arnst	General surgery clinic consultation
M-71	Jena Sage DeLeon	Orthopedic clinic followup note
M-73	Mary Margaret Kalter	Vascular surgery clinic consultation
M-74	Rudy Briones	General surgery consultation
M-78	Wayne M. Emerson	Orthopedic clinic followup note
M-79	Margaret Barger	Hematology/Oncology clinic followup note

M-80	James Sebastian Wright	Internal medicine clinic followup
M-83	Maria Irene Flores	Orthopedic clinic preop history & physical
M-85	Barbara Ann Tinka	Hematology/Oncology clinic followup note
M-88	Roseanne Erickson	Internal medicine initial visit
M-89	Patrick Joseph Flynn	Orthopedics shoulder clinic consultation
M-91	Rosemary George	Internal medicine clinic followup note
M-92	Tracy M. Dooley	Orthopedic spine clinic followup note
M-94	Paul DuBose	Internal medicine geriatrics clinic followup note
M-95	Jimmy Wu	Orthopedic clinic followup note
M-97	Oma Gaye Enderle	Internal medicine clinic followup note
M-99	Bernadette Dolly	Orthopedic spine clinic followup note

GLOSSARY OF KEY TERMS

N.B.: Brief definitions are given here; see unabridged English or medical dictionary for full and complete definitions.

abstractor   one who creates an abstract or summary; for example, one who abstracts a medical record

American Association for Medical Transcription (AAMT)   first international professional association for medical transcriptionists, formed in 1978

American Health Information Management Association (AHIMA)   professional organization for Health Information Management (HIM) professionals

American Medical Association (AMA)   professional organization for physicians

apprenticeship   training of a specific trade or craft incorporating both hands-on experience working with a skilled worker and related classroom instruction

assimilation   the process of receiving new facts or responding to new situations in conformity with what is already known

Association for Healthcare Documentation Integrity (AHDI)   name change adopted for AAMT in 2007 in order to include a more broad array of healthcare documentation professionals; for example, not only medical transcriptionists but also medical editors, abstractors, voice recognition editors, speech recognition editors

auditor   one who is authorized to examine and verify accounts, as in a Joint Committee audit

automated speech recognition (ASR)   software that allows the spoken word to be recorded by a speech engine, thereby automatically creating a medical record that is subject to medical editing

back-end speech recognition technology   the actual speech-to-text conversion takes place *after* the speaker has dictated

block format   letter style in which the entire letter is justified left and single-spaced, except for double spacing between paragraphs

blueprint domains   stated areas of content outlined that assess knowledge and skills on the RHDS and CHDS examinations

carpal tunnel syndrome   nerve entrapment characterized by pain, numbness, and tingling; often seen in those who overuse their hands

CECs   continuing education credits, usually awarded on an hour-by-hour basis; for example, a two-hour lecture would qualify for 2 CECs

Certified Healthcare Documentation Specialist (CHDS)   one who has taken and passed the certifying exam given by AHDI after this credential was rebranded in June 2013 and includes an expanded level 2 healthcare documentation skill set not previously evaluated on prior CMT exams

Certified Medical Transcriptionist (CMT)   one who has taken and passed the certifying exam given by AHDI prior to June 2013 and possesses and meets the minimum skill set needed to work as a level 2 medical transcriptionist

cleft palate   a birth defect resulting in an opening or cleft in the roof of the mouth; congenital fissure of the roof of the mouth

Clinical Document Architecture (CDA)   a Health Level Seven (HL7) standard that provides a framework for the encoding, formatting and semantics of electronic documents

Clinical Documentation Industry Association (CDIA)   formerly a not-for-profit trade association representing the management and delivery of clinical documentation services (this association closed down in April 2012)

contextual content   referring to the content in regard to where a medical editor is working in a particular report; e.g., "PCP" can refer to primary care physician in the context of demographics or the beginning of a report, it can refer to a patient care plan in the context of a discharge summary, or it can refer to pulmonary capillary pressure in the context of the respiratory system or the laboratory data

continuous speech recognition (CSR) another name for speech recognition

Credential Qualifying Examination (CQE) combination of two exams, the RHDS and the CHDS exams, given by AHDI in one sitting instead of taking each exam separately, for qualified candidates

database a large collection of data organized especially for rapid search and retrieval, as by a computer

dictator profiles for the purposes of this text, this refers to the specific style in which healthcare providers (including healthcare providers with accents) dictate medical records; each has distinct phraseology and terminology

draft document first draft of a document; a document that has not been edited or proofread

diphthong a gliding monosyllabic speech sound, as in the "th" sound

end user the ultimate consumer of a finished product, such as a medical record

English-as-a-second-language (ESL) those for whom English is not the first language; usually those who immigrated to this country

EVRT electronic voice recognition translation, which is software for translating vocal sounds

externship a learning opportunity to experience the workplace and explore a career opportunity

flag (a report) to mark a transcribed document to indicate a perceived problem with the dictation

front-end speech recognition technology with this method, the actual speech-to-text conversion takes place while the speaker is dictating, *concurrently*

healthcare documentation specialist (HDS) a trained professional who types (transcribes or keyboards) original medical reports while listening to medical dictation

health information management (HIM) working with and managing information in the healthcare industry

Health Information and Management Systems Society (HIMSS) a global, cause-based, not-for-profit organization focused on better health through information technology

Health Level Seven (HL7) Health Level Seven is a standard for exchanging information between medical applications; this standard defines a format for the transmission of health-related information

Health Story Project (HSP) the purpose of this project was to create standard "templates" for the common document types (H&P, Consultation Note, Progress Note, Procedure Note, Discharge Summary) using an HL7 standard called Clinical Document Architecture (CDA)

healthcare documentation specialist umbrella term coined by AHDI for medical transcriptionists, medical editors, and others who work in the healthcare documentation arena

high reliability ways of maintaining consistently high levels of safety and quality over time and across all healthcare services and settings; this model outlines three requirements for achieving high reliability: (1) leadership, (2) safety culture, and (3) robust process improvement

hearing acuity refers to the keenness or sharpness of hearing

homonyms one of two or more words spelled and pronounced alike but different in meaning, as in the noun quail (bird) and the verb quail (to wither or decline)

homophones one of two or more words pronounced alike but different in spelling and meaning, as in the words to, too, and two

internship an opportunity to work at a company for a designated period of time as a method of on-the-job training

intonation manner of utterance; the rise and fall in pitch of the voice in speech

intramuscular within the muscle tissue

intrathecal within the spinal canal

job classification the act or process of assigning jobs to categories or groups according to established criteria

learned dictation or learned language reference to how speech recognition equipment "learns" dictators' voices, phraseology, and styles of dictation

lisp a speech defect in which sibilants (the "s" and "z" sounds) are pronounced as "th"

macros a series of commands and actions used to automate tasks routinely performed; in transcription, this is commonly known as a program that expands words, phrases, paragraphs, report templates, and so on; e.g., an entry—and thus the keying in—of "pt" could be set to expand to "patient," an entry of "hx" could be set to expand to "history," and an entry of "T" could be set to expand to "temperature"

medical editor or medical editing (ME) an HDS (with training) who reads along while listening to medical dictation, making editorial corrections to a medical record

medical transcriptionist (MT) a trained professional who types (transcribes or keyboards) original medical reports while listening to medical dictation

medical transcription service organization (MTSO) companies that employ healthcare documentation specialists

mnemonics a technique of improving the memory, as in mnemonic device

modified block format letter style in which the sender's and recipient's addresses and the body of the letter are justified left, but the date and closing are tabbed to the center of the page

negative contractions verb combination of "is not" or "will not," into "isn't" or "won't"

networking the cultivation of productive relationships for employment or business; the establishment of a computer network

over-editing continuing to edit a medical report, even though the changes have no effect on accuracy or meaning; overly zealous editing

phonetics the study and systemic classification of the sounds made in spoken utterance (language)

proctored examination an examination during which a person (proctor) is physically present, overseeing the entire event

professional association accredited group that people join for the benefit of learning about their chosen career field, for networking benefits, for earning CECs

proprietary platforms or programs software that is owned by an individual or a company (usually the one that developed it); major restrictions are involved with its use, including a *source code* that is almost always kept secret

quality assurance (QA) a person or a department where "flagged" reports are sent for clarification and correction; a person or department where reports are routinely proofread for quality and accuracy with feedback given to employees on a regular basis

Registered Healthcare Documentation Specialist (RHDS) one who has taken and passed the RHDS exam administered by AHDI after this credential was rebranded in June 2013 and includes an expanded level 1 healthcare documentation skill set not previously evaluated on prior RMT exams

Registered Medical Transcriptionist (RMT) one who has taken and passed the RMT exam administered by AHDI prior to June 2013 and possesses and meets the minimum skill set needed to work as a level 1 medical transcriptionist

real-time refers to at this exact day and time

regulatory agencies private, non-profit, or governmental bodies with the authority and purpose of bringing safety, order, and uniformity to the healthcare industry (and others) for a fee

repetitive-use injury damage caused to the body by overuse of one or more of its parts; see carpal tunnel syndrome

return on investment (ROI) the concept of an investment of some resource yielding a benefit to the investor

rhythm an ordered, recurrent alteration of strong and weak elements in the flow of sound and silence in speech

semi-block format letter style similar to the modified block format, except that each paragraph is indented instead of flush left

sentinel event an unexpected death or serious physical injury—including loss of limb or function—or psychological injury, or the risk thereof

speech recognition engine the speech recognition engine is the software's ability to "learn" speech patterns as medical records are dictated into it; these can be learned correctly or incorrectly

speech recognition editor (SRE) an HDS (with training) who reads along while listening to medical dictation, making editorial corrections to a medical record; same as medical editor

speech recognition technology (SRT) speech recognition (SR) is the translation of spoken words into text; it is also known as "automatic speech recognition" (ASR), "computer speech recognition," or just "speech to text" (STT)

straight transcription referring to typing (transcribing or keyboarding) medical reports while listening to dictation as opposed to medical editing

stress to emphasize, as to accent a syllable; intense effort or exertion; strain or pressure

stuttering   speech disorder that includes speaking with involuntary disruption or blocking of speech with spasmodic repetition

sublingual   under the tongue

The Joint Commission (TJC)   an independent not-for-profit organization that evaluates and accredits healthcare organizations and programs in this country

track changes   the track changes function in Microsoft Word allows the medical editor to keep a record of changes made to a document; a useful tool in managing changes made by several reviewers, for QA auditors, and in a teaching or training situation (*after track changes are accepted or rejected, final copies should be checked once more for incidental spacing errors and such that may have been erroneously retained*)

traditional transcription   interchangeable with "straight" transcription

transdermal   to absorb through the skin into the blood stream

verbatim   word-for-word; following the exact words

vested interest   personal or private reason for wanting something to be done or to happen

vocal polyps or nodules   mass of tissue, perhaps a lymph node, that bulges or projects outward or upward from the normal surface level of the vocal cord (voice box)

voice recognition editor (VRE)   an HDS (with training) who reads along while listening to medical dictation, making editorial corrections to a medical record; same as medical editor

voice recognition engine   the voice recognition engine is the software's ability to "learn" speech patterns as medical records are dictated into it; these can be learned correctly or incorrectly

"word salad"   slang referring to the jumble of words that can occasionally result from speech recognition equipment aberrations

APPENDICES

APPENDIX A: NAMES OF DICTATING HEALTHCARE PROFESSIONALS

Last Name	First Name	Specialty	Accent
Aaron, DO	Marie	Family Practice	*
Altman, MD	Robert	Pulmonary Surgery/Respiratory Medicine	*
Andrew, MD	Lynne	Internal Medicine	*
Avalon, MD	Carl Erickson	Anesthesiology	*
Baker, MD	Michael	Physical Medicine and Rehabilitation	*
Barton, FNP	Rebecca	Family Nurse Practitioner	Texan
Basswood, MD	Anne	Neurology	*
Bautista, MD	Carlos	Physical Medicine and Rehabilitation	*
Brian, MD	Beth	Infectious Disease	*
Bruckman, MD	Grayson	Radiology	British
Bumbak, MD	Rosemary	Obstetrics/Gynecology	*
Castillo, MD	David	Orthopedic Surgery	*
Cohen, MD	David H.	Hematology/Oncology	*
Cole, MD	Elizabeth	Pediatric Urology	*
Collins, RHIA	Katherine	Director, HIM Department	Texan
Connerly, MD	Antonia	Pediatrics	*
Craven, MD	Margaret	Orthopedic Shoulder Surgery	Northeastern
Daily, MD	Jon Kyle	Oromaxillofacial Surgery	*
Dale, MD	Wanda P.	Neurosurgery	*
Delaney, MD	Chuck	Anesthesiology	*
Dickinson, PhD	Stella Rose	Psychology/Social Services	*
Dodd, MD	Carol	Orthopedic Surgery	*
Dugan, MD	Joan	Orthopedic Knee Surgery	Northeastern
Easterly, MD	Diana L.	Pediatric Neurology	*
Eaton, MD	Martha C.	Family Practice/Geriatrics	*
Ernest, MD	Samuel	Emergency Department	Northeastern
Erwin, MD	L. Willem	Radiation Oncology	German
Fields, MD	Gilbert M.	Orthopedic Surgery	Northeastern
Fisher, MD	Solomon T.	Hematology/Oncology	Northeastern
Fractor, MT	Jann	Radiology/Mammography Technician	*
Fry, MD	Danila R.	Plastic Surgery	Russian
Galbraith, FNP	Linda	Family Nurse Practitioner	*
Garcia, MD	John G.	Neurology	*
Gatlin, MD	Joshua Stephen	Pulmonology	*
Gerard, DO	Michael	Obstetrics/Gynecology	*
Gonzales, PhD	Cynthia G.	Psychology/Social Services	*

Last Name	First Name	Specialty	Accent
Gordon, MD	Stephen C.	Hematology/Oncology	*
Gromeko, MD	Anya	Orthopedic Surgery	Russian
Hampton, MD	Faye	Rheumatology	*
Haskill, MD	Mark L.	Orthopedic Surgery	*
Haskill, MD	Maura L.	Orthopedic Ankle Surgery	Northeastern
Iaccarino, RN	Anna Maria	Scrub Nurse	*
Jackson, MD	Toni	Cardiology	*
Jett, RN	Jimmy Dale	Circulating Nurse	*
Johnson, DDS	Robert P.	Dental Surgery	*
Jordan, MD	Trevor	Nephrology	*
Keathley, MD	Patrick	Endocrinology	*
Kelly, MD	Dana	Urology	*
Kester, MD	Bernard	General Surgery	*
King, MD	T. Washington	Neurology	*
Kingston, DO	Linda L.	Family Practice	*
Kofos, MD	Patricia	Pediatric Intensivist	*
Lanewala, MD	David	Orthopedic Surgery	*
Lawrence, MD	Nancy	Internal Medicine	*
Lee, MD	Howard H.	Orthopedic Surgery	*
Lopez, MD	Eric J.	Oncology	*
Loyd, MD	Sherman	Internal Medicine	*
Luken, CMT, AHDI-F	Kristine Anne	BES Program Coordinator	Northeastern
Mayoral, MD	Jesus	Colorectal Surgery/Pelvic Floor Medicine	*
McClure Jr, MD	James A.	General Surgery/Colorectal Surgery	Midwestern
McGinness, MD	Susan	Family Practice	*
Medina, MD	Leon	Internal Medicine	*
Mendesz, MD	Charles	Urology Surgery/Nephrology	Hispanic
Miller, MD	Ken	Gastroenterology	*
Moffett, MD	Michel	ENT/Oral Surgery	*
Montfort, MD	William	Cardiology	Irish
Mooney, MD	Jean W.	Internal Medicine	Northeastern
Moore, JD	Martha C.	Attorney	*
Morris	Mary Graham	Quality Assurance Supervisor	Texan
Mosbacker, MD	Luke	Rheumatology Clinic	*
Murray, MD	George	Interventional Radiology	Irish
Naimi, MD	Yasmin	Ophthalmology	Middle Eastern
Okano, MD	Midori	Ophthalmology	*
Oswalt, MD	Savant	Hematology/Oncology	*
Panagides, MD	Michael	Internal Medicine/Nephrology	Greek
Patel, MD	L. Prasad	General Surgery	Indian

Last Name	First Name	Specialty	Accent
Patrick, MD	Lucinda	Internal Medicine	*
Pavari, MD	Leela	Oromaxillofacial Surgery	Indian
Pavari, MD	Raj	Orthopedics	Indian
Peebles, MD	Sandra	Internal Medicine	*
Phillips, MD	Reed	Pediatrics	*
Phipps, MD	Anderson	Family Medicine/Geriatrics	*
Pittfield, MD	Leah	Otorhinolaryngology	*
Reardon, DO	Ronald	Family Practice	*
Rhodes, MD	Yancy	Endocrinology	Scottish
Richards, MD	Don	Gastroenterology/Endoscopy	*
Risha, MD	Tillman	Obstetrics/Gynecology	Middle Eastern
Robertson, MD	Doris	Gastroenterology	*
Rodriguez, MD	Raquel	Orthopedic Surgery	Hispanic
Ruffolo, MD	Glenn	Hematology/Oncology	*
Russo, MD	David	General Surgery	*
Russo, MD	Holly	Neurosurgery	*
Salem, DO	Chris	Family Practice	*
Scott, MD	Charles W.	Obstetrics/Gynecology	*
Shaker, MD	Kenneth	Internal Medicine	*
Shuff, MD	Phyllis	Nephrology	*
Smith, MD	Jesse D.	Orthopedic Surgery	*
Stolga, MD	Mack	Trauma Surgery	*
Tabor, MD	Ly An	Vascular Surgery	Middle Eastern
Tew, MD	Charles	Nuclear Medicine	Chinese
Thompson, MD	Saul	Cardiology	*
Thorner, MD	Robin	Anesthesiology	*
Timmerman, MD	Callie	Dermatology	Northeastern
Tobar, MA	Rosalinda	Medical Assistant	Northeastern
Travis, MD	Murray	Obstetrics/Gynecology	*
Ventura, MD	Robert	Internal Medicine	*
Verlin, MD	Lloyd	Pulmonology	*
Wagner, PA-C	Jason	Orthopedics	*
Warren, MD	Tonya	Hematology/Oncology	*
Webb, MD	Zachary	Vascular Surgery	*
Wells, MD	A. Leigh	Internal Medicine	*
Wolfe, MD	Jeffrey	Cardiac Surgery	*
Youngblood, MD	Arnold R.	Neurosurgery	*
Zullig, MD	Jack	Orthopedic Surgery	*

* No dictation

APPENDIX B: CHALLENGING WORDS, TERMS, AND PREFIXES

Healthcare documentation specialists and medical editors must use critical thinking skills—listening carefully and considering the context—in editing medical dictation. Consider the following sound-alikes, their parts of speech, and the spelling of each.

N.B.: Brief definitions are used in this list; see an unabridged medical dictionary or English dictionary for complete definitions.

A

abduction—the act of drawing away from (often dictated "a-b-duction")

adduction—the act of drawing toward a center (often dictated "a-d-duction")

subduction—the act of drawing downward

aberration—deviation from the usual course or condition

abrasion—the wearing away of a substance or structure through some unusual or abnormal mechanical process

absorption—the soaking up of a substance by skin or other surface

adsorption—the adherence of a substance to a surface

acathexia—the inability to retain bodily secretions

cachexia—a profound and marked state of constitutional disorder

afferent—carrying impulses *toward* a center or part

efferent—carrying *away* from a central organ or part

allograft—transfers or transplants between two individuals of the same species

autograft—transfers or transplants from the same person

anuresis—retention of urine within the bladder

enuresis—urinary incontinence

aphagia—inability to swallow

aphasia—absent or impaired comprehension or communication by speech or writing— may be transient, as in acquired lesion or swelling of the brain

apophysis—outgrowth or swelling

epiphysis—a center for formation of bone substance at each extremity of long bones

areola—**(n)** a circular area of a different color surrounding a central point, as in the breast

areolae—plural of areola

areolar—**(adj)** pertaining to or containing areolae

arrhythmia—irregular heartbeat

eurhythmia—regular pulse

arteriosclerosis—a group of diseases characterized by thickening and the loss of elasticity of arterial walls

atherosclerosis—hardening of the arteries caused by the deposition of calcium and cholesterol in the arterial walls

arteriostenosis—ossification of an artery

arteriotomy—surgical opening of an artery

arteritis—inflammation of artery

arthritis—inflammation of a joint

arterial—pertaining to one or more arteries

arteriole—a small arterial branch

arthropathy—any joint disease

arthroplasty—plastic surgery of a joint

aura—**(n)** subjective evidence of the beginning of either a seizure-like episode or a migraine headache

aural—pertaining to the ears or to an aura

oral—pertaining to the mouth

B

basil—**(n)** an herb, a seasoning

basal—**(adj)** basal ganglia, basal cell, basal metabolic rate

bronchi—plural of bronchus

rhonchi—pertaining to a rattling in the throat or a dry, coarse rale in the bronchial tubes

buccal—**(adj)** describing mucosa inside cheek, as in buccal cavity, buccal smear

buckle—(ophthalmology) surgical repair of retinal tears, as in scleral buckle procedure; (orthopedics) buckle fracture of phalanx, wire-fixation buckle

bursa—**(n)** a sac or sac-like cavity filled with viscid fluid

bursae—plural of bursa

C

calculous—**(adj)** pertaining to, of the nature of, or affected with calculus

calculus—**(n)** a hard, pebble-like mass formed within the body, as in the gallbladder

callous—**(adj)** unfeeling; the adjective form of callus

callus—**(n)** a callosity

cancellous—**(adj)** of a reticular, spongy, or lattice-like structure; said mainly of bony tissue

cancellus—**(n)** any structure arranged like a lattice

canker—ulceration, primarily of the mouth and lips

chancre—the primary lesion of syphilis

cerebellum—that part of the brain behind the cerebrum

cerebrum—the main portion of the brain

chordae—plural of chorda, as in chordae tendineae (heart)

chordee—associated with hypospadias (downward bowing of the penis)

cirrhosis—a progressive disease in which healthy liver tissue is replaced with scar tissue, thereby preventing the liver from functioning properly

xerosis—abnormal dryness, as of the eye, skin, or mouth

sclerosis—hardening, as hardening of a body part from inflammation

cite—**(v)** to quote

site—**(n)** a location

sight—the function of seeing; a view, or to take aim

colectomy—excision of a portion of the colon

colpectomy—excision of the vagina

colonic—pertaining to the colon

clonic—pertaining to muscular contractions and relaxations that alternate in rapid succession; tonic-clonic seizures

cornea—**(n)** the transparent structure forming the anterior part of the sclera of the eye, i.e., cornea of the eye

corneal—**(adj)** resembling the cornea of the eye

cornua—**(n)** pl. of cornu, a structure resembling a horn in shape, i.e., cornua uteri

cystoscopy—direct visual examination of the urinary tract with a cystoscope

cystostomy—the formation of an opening into the bladder

cystotomy—surgical incision of the urinary bladder

D

diffuse—**(adj)** scattered, not localized; e.g., diffuse infiltrates

defuse—**(v)** to make a situation less harmful; to calm a crisis

dilation—the act of being dilated or stretched

dilatation—condition of being stretched beyond the normal dimensions

diuresis—an increased secretion of urine

uresis—the passage of urine

dysphagia—difficulty in swallowing

dysphasia—impairment of speech

dysplasia—abnormality of development

E

effusion—escape of a fluid into a part

affusion—pouring of water upon the body to reduce temperature

infusion—continuous introduction of solution, especially into a vein

emphysema—a pathological accumulation of air in tissues or organs, as in the lungs

empyema—accumulation of pus in a cavity

enervation—lack of nervous energy

innervation—the supply of nervous energy or of nerve stimulus sent to a part

enterocleisis—closure of a wound in the intestine

enteroclysis—the injection of a nutrient or medicinal liquid into the bowel

epididymis—a cord-like structure attached to the back of the testis

epididymitis—inflammation of the epididymis

exostosis—a bony growth that emanates from the surface of a bone

enostosis—an osseous tumor within the cavity of a bone

expiration—synonym for death; breathing out or exhalation

extirpation—to remove entirely; as in extirpation of varicose veins

extubation—to remove a tube, as a nasogastric tube, from a patient

F

facial—pertaining to the face

fascial—pertaining to the fascia (a layer of fibrous tissue)

facioplasty—plastic surgery of the face

fascioplasty—plastic surgery on a fascia

fascicular—pertaining to a fascicle

vesicular—composed of or relating to small, sac-like bodies

testicular—pertaining to a testis

facies—pertaining to the anterior or ventral aspect of the head from forehead to chin

feces—the excrement discharged from the intestines

fascicle—a small bundle, like muscle or nerve fibers

vesicle—any small bladder or sac containing liquid

vesical—pertaining to the urinary bladder

fecal—pertaining to excrement discharged from the intestines

thecal—pertaining to an enclosing case or sheath

fossa—a trench or channel; a general term for a hollow or depressed area

fossae—plural of fossa

fundus—the bottom or base

fungus—a vegetable cellular organism that subsists on organic matter—a mushroom is a fungus

G

gait—(n) a manner of walking or moving on foot

gate—(n) an opening in a wall or a fence

glans—(n, singular) a small, rounded mass of gland-like body; e.g., end of penis

gland(s)—(n) aggregation of cells specialized to secrete or excrete; e.g., adrenal gland, ciliary glands, Skene gland, Tyson glands

Glidewire—(trade name) Glidewire catheter, Glidewire Gold surgical guidewire

guidewire—(generic) surgical equipment; e.g., cannula with preloaded guidewire, catheter guidewire, floppy guidewire, silk guidewire, steerable guidewire

graft—(n) tissue for implantation (grafting)

graph—(n) a written record, diagram

grasp—(v) grab hold of or seize, as with a surgical instrument

H

heels—(n) parts of the feet (hindfoot)

heals—(v) the process of curing an illness, restoring to health

hemithorax—one side of the chest

hemothorax—a collection of blood in the pleural cavity

pneumothorax—accumulation of air or gas in the pleural space

hemostasis—the arrest of bleeding

homeostasis—a tendency to stability in the normal body states of an organism

hyperglycemia—abnormally increased content of sugar in the blood

hyperglycinemia—heredity disorder involving excessive glycine in the blood

hypoglycemia—abnormally low content of sugar in the blood

hypertension—persistently high arterial blood pressure

hypotension—abnormally low blood pressure

I

ileum—part of the small intestine (gastrointestinal system)

ilium—part of the pelvis (musculoskeletal system)

ileus—disease (obstruction of the small intestine)

in situ—in its normal place, confined to the site of origin

in toto—totally

in vivo—within the living body

in vitro—within a test tube (glass)

K

ketosis—a condition characterized by an abnormally elevated concentration of ketone bodies in the body tissues and fluids

keratosis—a horny growth

L

legion—group of soldiers, as in a "legion of men prepared to attack"

lesion—a sore on the body, as in "the facial lesion was red and painful"

loop—an instrument used to grasp and remove the lens; "lens loop"

loupe—a pair of glasses worn by a surgeon; "loupe magnification"

M

malleolus—a bone of the ankle

malleus—a bone of the ear

mammaplasty or **mammoplasty**—plastic reconstruction of the breast

mammillaplasty—plastic surgery of the nipple and areola

metacarpal—relating to the hand

metatarsal—relating to the foot, between the instep and the toes

mucosa—**(n)** a mucous membrane

mucosal—**(adj)** pertaining to the mucous membrane

mucous—**(adj)** pertaining to or resembling mucus

mucus—**(n)** secretion or slime of the mucous membrane

myelitis—inflammation of the spinal cord

myositis—inflammation of a voluntary muscle

N

naris—the nostril; one side of the nasal opening

nares—plural of naris; both nasal openings

nephritis—inflammation of a kidney

neuritis—inflammation of a nerve

nuchal—the back, nape, or scruff of the neck

knuckle—the dorsal aspect of any phalangeal joint

O

orthopaedics or **orthopedics**—interchangeable; referring to the branch of medicine concerned with the correction or prevention of skeletal deformities, disorders, or injuries; *N.B.*: the spelling "orthopedics" is used exclusively in *Quality Medical Editing*

ostial—relating to any orifice, or ostium

osteal—bony

P

palate—the partition separating the nasal and oral cavities

palliate—to reduce the severity of, to relieve

palpation—the act of feeling with the hand

palpitation—unduly rapid action of the heart

para—combining form meaning beside, near, past, beyond, the opposite, abnormal

peri—prefix meaning around or about

pericardial—**(adj)** pertaining to the membrane surrounding the heart and great vessels

pericardium—**(n)** the membrane surrounding the heart

perineal—pertaining to the perineum, or genital region

peritoneal—pertaining to the peritoneum, or membrane lining the abdominal wall

peroneal—pertaining to the fibula, or the outer side of the leg

peritoneum—the serous membrane lining the abdominopelvic walls

perineum—the pelvic floor and the associated structures occupying the pelvic outlet

plain x-ray—no contrast media was used; a noncontrast film

plane x-ray—a tomogram

pleural space—space between the parietal and visceral layers of the pleura

plural space—more than one space

precordial—pertaining to the region over the heart and lower part of the thorax

precordium—the region of the thorax immediately over the heart

psittacosis—an infectious disease of parrots and other birds that may be transmitted to humans

psychosis—a general term for any major mental disorder of organic or emotional origin

sycosis—a disease marked by inflammation of the hair follicles

R

radical—directed to the cause; directed to the root or source of a morbid process

radicle—any one of the smallest branches of a vessel or nerve

reflux—a backward flow

reflex—an involuntary response to a stimulus

S

scirrhous—**(adj)** pertaining to a cancer that is stony hard to the touch

scirrhus—**(n)** a hard cancerous growth, as in scirrhous carcinoma

serious—said or done in earnest; sincere

supination—the act of rotating the arm so that the palm of the hand is forward or upward

suppuration—the formation or discharge of pus

T

tendinous—resembling a tendon

tendinitis—inflammation of a tendon or tendons

track—**(n)** a path or groove, as in a needle track or a railroad track

tract—**(n)** system of body parts, as in the digestive tract, the respiratory tract; a bundle of nerve fibers having a common origin, termination, and function

U

ureter—**(n)** tube through which urine travels to the bladder—we have a left and a right ureter

urethra—**(n)** a membranous canal through which urine travels from the bladder to the surface—we have one urethra

ureteral—pertaining to the ureters

urethral—pertaining to the urethra

V

vena cava—**(singular)** one of two venae cavae, superior or inferior

venae cavae—**(plural)** the two largest veins in the body

vesical—pertaining to the urinary bladder

vesicle—any small bladder or sac containing liquid

fascicle—a small bundle, like muscle or nerve fibers

villous—**(adj)** shaggy with soft hairs; covered with villi

villus—**(n)** a small vascular process or protrusion

viral—pertaining to a virus

virile—possessing masculine traits

W

weather—**(n)** the climate, the atmosphere; e.g., under the weather

whether—**(conj)** used as a function word usually with "or"; e.g., whether black or white, whether he is alive or dead, whether to come or to go

womb—the uterus

wound—trauma to the body

APPENDIX C: DRUG LIST: BRAND NAMES WITH CORRESPONDING GENERIC TERMS

Brand name or trade name drugs are transcribed using an initial capital letter (initial cap). The generic equivalent is typed in all lower case. Healthcare documentation specialists and medical editors usually have an up-to-date drug book as part of their reference material, i.e., published within the last two years.

The partial list of drugs below shows each brand name followed by the generic name, then a brief descriptor. Not every generic drug has an equivalent brand name. Also, there is what is known as "off-label" uses for drugs, e.g., they may be used for conditions they were not originally intended to treat. One example of this is methotrexate, a common antineoplastic agent or cancer drug, which in some instances may be prescribed to patients with multiple sclerosis, severe rheumatoid arthritis, or severe psoriasis.

N.B.: The drugs and terms used in this list are often dictated in medical reports. We offer abbreviated definitions here. Please see a medical dictionary, a recently published drug reference book, or check online sources such as http://www.drugs.com or http://www.rxlist.com for more information on each one.

A

Accupril—(generic quinapril) used to treat hypertension and heart failure

Actos—(generic pioglitazone) an antidiabetic agent used to treat type 2 diabetes mellitus

Adderall and Adderall XR—(generic dextroamphetamine and amphetamine) used to treat attention-deficit/hyperactivity disorder (ADHD) and narcolepsy, which are recurrent, brief, uncontrollable episodes of sleep

Advair and Advair HFA—(generic fluticasone and salmeterol) a corticosteroid used to treat asthma and COPD

Afinitor—(generic everolimus) antineoplastic agent used in the treatment of advanced renal cell cancer

albuterol—generic drug used to treat or prevent exercise-induced bronchospasm in patients with COPD

Aldactone—(generic spironolactone) a diuretic used to manage edema

Aldara—(generic imiquimod) used to treat external genital and perianal warts, superficial basal cell carcinoma, and actinic keratosis on face or scalp

Allegra, Allegra-D, Allegra-D 24 Hour, and Allegra ODT—(generic fexofenadine) an antihistamine used to treat seasonal allergic rhinitis and chronic urticaria

Ambien and Ambien CR—(generic zolpidem) used in the treatment of short-term insomnia

Apo-Prednisone—(generic prednisone) corticosteroid used in the treatment of rheumatoid arthritis, autoimmune disorders, and in a variety of other conditions; this drug is available in a variety of brand names

Apo-Terazosin—(generic terazosin) used in the management of mild to moderate hypertension

Apo-Trazodone—(generic trazodone) an antidepressant used to treat major depressive disorders

Arava—(generic leflunomide) used to treat active rheumatoid arthritis

Arimidex—(generic anastrozole) an antineoplastic agent used to treat breast cancer

Arixtra—(generic fondaparinux) used to prevent deep vein thrombosis (DVT) prior to surgery

Arthrotec—(generic diclofenac and misoprostol) used in the treatment of osteoarthritis and rheumatoid arthritis in patients at high risk for NSAID-induced gastric and duodenal ulceration

ASA—(generic aspirin) acetyl salicylic acid

Ativan—(generic lorazepam) used to manage anxiety disorders

Atrovent and Atrovent HFA—(generic ipratropium) used to relieve rhinorrhea and rhinitis

Avapro—(generic irbesartan) used to treat hypertension and diabetic neuropathy

Azulfidine and Azulfidine EN-tabs—(generic sulfasalazine) used in the treatment of rheumatoid arthritis and ulcerative colitis

B

BCG—(bacillus Calmette-Guerin) BCG live is used intravesically for treatment and prophylaxis following transurethral resection; BCG vaccine is used as immunization against Mycobacterium tuberculosis

Betadine—(generic povidone-iodine) a topical antiseptic used externally for the prevention of topical infections related to surgery, burns, minor cuts or scrapes

Betapace and Betapace AF—(generic sotalol) an antiarrhythmic used to maintain normal sinus rhythm in patients with atrial fibrillation and atrial flutter

Bicitra—(generic citric acid and sodium nitrate combination) used to keep urine alkaline to prevent kidney stones

Boniva—(generic ibandronate) used in the treatment and prevention of osteoporosis

Botox—(generic onabotulinumtoxinA or botulinum toxin type A) treatment of strabismus and blepharospasm associated with dystonia, used for multiple other medical purposes in children and adults

Buspirex—(generic buspirone) an antianxiety agent used to manage generalized anxiety disorder

C

Cardizem, Cardizem CD, Cardizem LA, and Cardizem SR—(generic diltiazem) used to treat essential hypertension, angina, atrial fibrillation or atrial flutter, and paroxysmal supraventricular tachycardia (PSVT)

Casodex—(generic bicalutamide) used in patients with metastatic prostate cancer

cefazolin—generic drug used to treat respiratory tract, skin, genital, urinary tract, biliary tract, bone and joint infections. No brand names are listed for this product.

Celebrex—(generic celecoxib) an NSAID used in the management of acute pain

Celestone—(generic betamethasone) a semisynthetic glucocorticoid with antiinflammatory effects and toxicity similar to those of cortisol

Cipro, Cipro XL, and Cipro XR—(generic ciprofloxacin) an antibiotic used mainly to treat urinary tract infections

Cleocin HCl and Cleocin T—(generic clindamycin) Cleocin in either form is an antibiotic skin product for treatment of bacterial infections and is offered in a variety of brand names; Cleocin HCl is administered orally; Cleocin T can be administered topically or vaginally

Claforan—(generic cefotaxime) a cephalosporin antibiotic used to treat susceptible infections in respiratory tract, skin, bone and joint, urinary tract, and gynecologic; active against many penicillin-resistant pneumococci

Clinoril—(generic sulindac) an NSAID used in the management of inflammatory diseases including osteoarthritis, rheumatoid arthritis, bursitis, tendinitis, painful shoulder

Codeine Contin—(generic codeine) a narcotic used to treat mild to moderate pain

Colace—(generic docusate) an over-thecounter (OTC) stool softener

Colcrys—(generic colchicine) an antigout agent used in the prevention and treatment of acute flares of gout

Coreg and Coreg CR—(generic carvedilol) used in patients with mild to severe heart failure

Coumadin—(generic warfarin) anticoagulant used as a prophylaxis and treatment of thromboembolic disorders and embolic complications, e.g., recurrent myocardial infarction, stroke

Cymbalta—(generic duloxetine) used in the treatment of major depressive disorder

D

Depakote, Depakote ER, and Depakote Sprinkles—(generic divalproex sodium) an anticonvulsant used in the treatment of multiple seizure types

Depo-Medrol—(generic methylprednisolone) used primarily as an anti-inflammatory or immunosuppressant agent in the treatment of a variety of diseases, including autoimmune origin; also, prevention and treatment of graft-versus-host disease following bone marrow transplantation

Detrol and Detrol LA—(generic tolterodine) used to treat overactive bladder, urge incontinence

Dexasone and Dexasone LA—(generic dexamethasone) a corticosteroid used as an anti-inflammatory agent

Dexilant—(generic dexlansoprazole) short-term (four-week) treatment for heartburn associated with GERD; short-term (eight-week) treatment of all grades of erosive esophagitis

Didrocal—(generic calcium carbonate and etidronate disodium) used in the treatment and prevention of postmenopausal osteoporosis and to prevent corticosteroid-induced osteoporosis

Dilantin—(generic phenytoin) used in the treatment of grand mal seizures and the prevention of seizures following head trauma

Diprivan—(generic propofol) general anesthetic

Drisdol—(generic ergocalciferol) a vitamin D dietary supplement used in the treatment of rickets, hypoparathyroidism, hypophosphatemia

Duragesic—(generic fentanyl) a narcotic transdermal patch used to treat chronic pain

Dyrenium—(generic triamterene) a diuretic used in the treatment of edema, hypertension

Dysport—(generic abobotulinumtoxinA) used to treat cervical dystonia (spasmodic torticollis); used for the temporary improvement in the appearance of lines or wrinkles of the face, for excessive sweating

E

Effexor and Effexor XR—(generic venlafaxine) used in the treatment of major depressive disorder, social anxiety disorder, panic disorder

Elixophyllin, Elixophyllin GG, and Elixophyllin KI—(generic theophylline) used in the treatment of reversible airway obstruction due to chronic asthma or other chronic lung diseases; theophylline is available under a variety of brand names

Enbrel—(generic etanercept) used in the treatment of psoriasis and rheumatoid arthritis

estradiol—generic drug, an estrogen derivative, used systemically to treat symptoms of menopause

F

Flexeril—(generic cyclobenzaprine) used as a muscle relaxant and to treat muscle spasms

Flomax—(generic tamsulosin) used in the treatment of benign prostatic hyperplasia (BPH)

Forteo—(generic teriparatide) used in the treatment of osteoporosis in women at high risk of fracture

Fosamax—(generic alendronate) used in the treatment and prevention of osteoporosis in postmenopausal females, also used in the treatment of Paget disease of the bone

G

Gen-Hydroxyurea—(generic hydroxyurea) an antineoplastic agent used in the treatment of melanoma, chronic ovarian cancer, and in sickle cell anemia

Garamycin (injection route)—(generic gentamicin systemic) an antibiotic normally used for gram-negative organisms, including respiratory tract infections, skin and soft tissue infections, abdominal and urinary tract infection, septicemia, and infective endocarditis

Glucotrol and Glucotrol XL—(generic glipizide) an oral antidiabetic agent used to manage type 2 diabetes mellitus

H

Hep-Lock, HepFlush-10—(generic heparin) an anticoagulant used in the prevention and treatment of thromboembolic disorders; as an anticoagulant for extracorporeal and dialysis procedures; heparin lock flush solution is intended only to maintain patency of IV devices and is **not** to be used for anticoagulant therapy

Hydrea—(generic hydroxyurea) an antineoplastic agent used in the treatment of melanoma, chronic myelocytic leukemia, ovarian cancer, and in sickle cell anemia (See Gen-Hydroxyurea listed previously)

I

Imuran—(generic azathioprine) an immunosuppressant agent used to prevent the rejection of kidney transplants and in the management of rheumatoid arthritis

K

Kenalog (topical)—(generic triamcinolone) a topical corticosteroid used in the treatment of oral inflammatory lesions and ulcerative lesions resulting from trauma

L

Lanoxin—(generic digoxin) an antiarrhythmic drug used to treat mild to moderate heart failure

Lasix—(generic furosemide) a loop diuretic (water pill) used to manage edema in patients with congestive heart failure (CHF), liver or kidney disease

Lexapro—(generic escitalopram) an antidepressant used to treat major depressive disorder

Lipitor—(generic atorvastatin) a statin drug that reduces the level of bad cholesterol (LDL) and triglycerides and increases the good cholesterol (HDL)

Lithobid—(generic lithium) antimanic agent used in the treatment of bipolar disorders

Lopressor—(generic metoprolol) beta blocker treatment of angina pectoris, hypertension, or hemodynamically stable acute myocardial infarction; this drug has a heightened risk of causing significant patient harm when used in error; significant differences exist between oral and IV dosing

Lopressor HCT—(generic metoprolol tartrate and hydrochlorothiazide) a combination of the beta blocker treatment of metoprolol and the diuretic treatment of hydrochlorothiazide to reduce edema

Lortab—(generic hydrocodone and acetaminophen) an opioid (narcotic) used in the treatment of moderate to severe pain

Lovenox—(generic enoxaparin) an anticoagulant used in unstable angina and to prevent deep vein thrombosis (DVT)

Lyrica—(generic pregabalin) used in the treatment of pain associated with diabetic peripheral neuropathy, partial-onset seizure disorder, management of fibromyalgia, postherpetic neuralgia

M

Macrobid—(generic nitrofurantoin) an antibiotic used to treat urinary tract infections

Mevacor—(generic lovastatin) a statin drug that reduces the level of bad cholesterol (LDL) and triglycerides and increases the good cholesterol (HDL)

Miacalcin—(generic calcitonin) a nasal spray used in the treatment of Paget disease and osteoporosis

Midol Extended Relief—(generic naproxen) analgesic, nonsteroidal anti-inflammatory drug (NSAID)

MiraLAX—(generic polyethylene glycol) used in the treatment of temporary constipation in adults

Mobic—(generic meloxicam) an NSAID used to treat osteoarthritis and rheumatoid arthritis

N

Neurontin—(generic gabapentin) an anticonvulsant used as adjunct treatment for epilepsy in adults and children age 12 or older and to treat partial seizures in children ages 3-12; also used in the management of postherpetic neuralgia in adults

Nexavar—(generic sorafenib) antineoplastic agent used in the treatment of liver cancer, thyroid cancer, and advanced renal cell cancer

Nexium—(generic esomeprazole) a proton pump inhibitor, used to treat gastroesophageal reflux disease (GERD)

Next Choice—(generic levonorgestrel) emergency contraceptive (birth control pill) following unprotected intercourse or possible contraceptive failure

Niaspan and Niaspan ER—(generic niacin) drug used to treat pancreatitis, hyperlipidemia, and to lower the risk of a myocardial infarction or heart attack

Nitro-Bid, Nitro-Dur, Nitro-Time, Nitrol, Nitrostat—(generic nitroglycerin) a vasodilator used to treat angina pectoris, congestive heart failure, and hypertension; used to relax and dilate the blood vessels, thus improving blood flow; this drug is available under a variety of brand names

Norvasc—(generic amlodipine) a calcium channel blocker used in the treatment of hypertension; this drug is available under a variety of brand names

Novo-Nortriptyline—(generic nortriptyline) a tricyclic antidepressant; this drug is available under a variety of brand names

NSAIDs—(dictated "en-saids") a category of drugs, nonsteroidal anti-inflammatory drugs, used to manage pain; available under a variety of both brand and generic names

NuvaRing—(generic ethinyl estradiol and etonogestrel) a vaginal ring used for contraception (birth control); insert ring and leave in place for three consecutive weeks, then remove for one week

O

Omnicef—(generic cefdinir) used to treat pneumonia, acute bacterial otitis media, acute exacerbations of chronic bronchitis, acute maxillary sinusitis, pharyngitis, tonsillitis, uncomplicated skin infections

OxyContin—(generic oxycodone) an opioid (narcotic), a controlled substance, used to treat moderate to severe pain; used for around-the-clock treatment of pain but not to be used on an "as-needed" basis

P

Paxil, Paxil CR—(generic paroxetine) a selective serotonin reuptake inhibitor (SSRI) antidepressant, used to treat major depressive disorder, panic disorder, obsessive compulsive disorder (OCD)

Plaquenil—(generic hydroxychloroquine) used in the suppression and treatment of acute attacks of malaria as well as the treatment of systemic lupus erythematosus (SLE) and rheumatoid arthritis

Plavix—(generic clopidogrel) an anticoagulant used to help prevent blood clots in patients with recent myocardial infarction, stroke, or peripheral artery disease

Plendil—(generic felodipine) a calcium channel blocker used in the treatment of hypertension

Pradaxa—(generic dabigatran etexilate) an anticoagulant used to prevent blood clots arising from atrial fibrillation, after cardiac valve replacement, after myocardial infarction, recurrent stroke

Prilosec—(generic omeprazole) used in the treatment of duodenal ulcer, gastric ulcer, heartburn, and other symptoms of GERD; this drug is available under a variety of brand names

Prinivil—(generic lisinopril) an angiotensin-converting enzyme (ACE) inhibitor used in the treatment of hypertension, congestive heart failure (CHF), and to improve survival after a heart attack

Prevacid—(generic lansoprazole) a proton pump inhibitor (PPI) used in the treatment of NSAID-associated gastric ulcers, active duodenal ulcers, erosive esophagitis, and GERD; this drug is available in several brand name forms and generic forms, some of which are bundled with other drugs, for example, lansoprazole and naproxen

Prolia—(generic denosumab) monoclonal antibody used to treat osteoporosis in postmenopausal females at high risk for fracture

Proscar—(generic finasteride) treatment of symptoms of benign prostatic hyperplasia (BPH) in males with an enlarged prostate

Provigil—(generic modafinil) central nervous system stimulant, a controlled substance, used to improve wakefulness in patients with narcolepsy, obstructive sleep apnea/hypopnea syndrome

R

Reclast—(generic zoledronic acid or zoledronate) oncology use—treatment of hypercalcemia of malignancy, multiple myeloma, bone metastases of solid tumors; non-oncology use—treating Paget disease of bone and osteoporosis in postmenopausal women and other uses

Reglan—(generic metoclopramide) gastrointestinal agent used to treat nausea and vomiting associated with chemotherapy or postsurgery; also short-term treatment of GERD in patients who have had no relief of symptoms with other medications

Relafen—(generic nabumetone) an NSAID used in the management of osteoarthritis and rheumatoid arthritis

Remeron—(generic mirtazapine) used in the treatment of major depressive disorders

Remicade—(generic infliximab) used in the treatment of rheumatoid arthritis, Crohn disease, ulcerative colitis, psoriasis, and a variety of other conditions

Renagel—(generic sevelamer) used to treat patients with chronic kidney disease on hemodialysis

Retrovir (generic zidovudine)—an antiviral agent used to treat HIV infection; also used to prevent maternal-to-fetal HIV transmission

Rheumatrex—(generic methotrexate) an antineoplastic agent used in the treatment of cancer; used also in the treatment of psoriasis and rheumatoid arthritis

Rituxan—(generic rituximab) an antineoplastic agent used to treat non-Hodgkin lymphoma or chronic lymphocytic leukemia as well as rheumatoid arthritis in combination with methotrexate

Robaxin—(generic methocarbamol) a skeletal muscle relaxant used to relieve muscle spasm associated with painful musculoskeletal conditions

Rocephin—(generic ceftriaxone) antibiotic used to treat bacterial infections such as lower respiratory tract infections, skin infections, meningitis, and a variety of other infections

S

Serax—(generic oxazepam) an anticonvulsant used to treat anxiety, ethanol withdrawal

Skelaxin—(generic metaxalone) skeletal muscle relaxant used to relieve acute, painful musculoskeletal conditions

Solu-Medrol—(generic methylprednisolone) a steroid used as an anti-inflammatory or immunosuppressant in the treatment of asthma, allergic reactions, flare-ups of illnesses, and variety of other medical problems; can also lessen some cancer symptoms; see Depo-Medrol previously noted

Synthroid—(generic levothyroxine) used as replacement or supplemental therapy in hypothyroidism

Synvisc—(generic hyaluronate and derivatives, hylan G-F 20) injectable fluid that acts as a lubricant and shock absorber for the joints of the knees; this drug is available under a variety of brand names

T

Tenormin—(generic atenolol) beta blocker used in the treatment of hypertension, management of angina, secondary prevention of postmyocardial infarction

Thrombate III—(antithrombin III [human] generic blood product derivative) used to prevent and treat thromboembolism in patients with hereditary antithrombin deficiency, particularly when undergoing obstetric or surgical procedures

Toprol-XL—(generic metoprolol) beta blocker treatment of angina pectoris, hypertension, or hemodynamically stable acute myocardial infarction; this drug has a heightened risk of causing significant patient harm when used in error; significant differences exist between oral and IV dosing

Trandate—(generic labetalol) beta blocker used to treat mild to severe hypertension

TriCor—(generic fenofibrate) brand name drug used in the treatment of elevated cholesterol and serum triglyceride levels

Tylox—(generic oxycodone and acetaminophen) a controlled narcotic used in the management of moderate to severe pain

U

Ultram—(generic tramadol) a narcotic-like pain reliever used in the treatment of moderate to severe pain

Ultradol—(generic etodolac) an NSAID used in the management of osteoarthritis, rheumatoid arthritis, and to manage acute pain (Utradol is the Canadian spelling)

V

Vancocin—(generic vancomycin) an antibiotic used to treat bacterial infections; indicated for the treatment of C difficile-associated diarrhea

Vicodin, Vicodin ES, Vicodin HP—(generic hydrocodone and acetaminophen) a controlled substance used in the treatment of moderate to severe pain

Voltaren (enteric-coated capsules) and Voltaren gel—(generic diclofenac) used in the treatment of osteoarthritis and rheumatoid arthritis in patients with a high risk of NSAID-induced gastric and duodenal ulcers

W

Wellbutrin, Wellbutrin SR, Wellbutrin XL—(generic bupropion) an antidepressant used in the treatment of major depressive disorders, including seasonal affective disorder (SAD)

X

Xanax, Xanax TS, Xanax XR—(generic alprazolam) a controlled substance used in the treatment of anxiety disorder, panic disorder associated with depression

Z

Zanaflex—(generic tizanidine) a short-term muscle relaxant used to treat muscle spasticity

Zantac—(generic ranitidine) used to prevent and treat GERD and ulcers in the stomach and intestines; this drug is available under a variety of brand names

Zaroxolyn—(generic metolazone) a diuretic, used in the management of edema, hypertension, congestive heart failure (CHF), and impaired renal function

Zemplar—(generic paricalcitol) a vitamin D analog used in the prevention and treatment of hyperparathyroidism associated with chronic kidney disease

Zocor—(generic simvastatin) cholesterol-lowering agent used to prevent strokes and heart attacks

Zoloft—(generic sertraline) an antidepressant used in the treatment of obsessive compulsive disorder (OCD), panic disorder, posttraumatic stress disorder (PTSD)

Zonegran—(generic zonisamide) an anticonvulsant used together with other anti-convulsant medications to treat partial seizures in adult epilepsy

Zosyn—(generic piperacillin and tazobactam sodium) penicillin antibiotic used to treat moderate to severe bacterial infections

Zyloprim—(generic allopurinol) reduces the production of uric acid in the body; used to treat gouty arthritis, kidney stones, nephropathy

APPENDIX D: THE OFFICIAL "DO NOT USE" LIST

In 2001, The Joint Commission issued a *Sentinel Event Alert* on the subject of medical abbreviations, and just one year later, its Board of Commissioners approved a National Patient Safety Goal requiring accredited organizations to develop and implement a list of abbreviations not to use. In 2004, The Joint Commission created its "do not use" list of abbreviations (see below) as part of the requirements for meeting that goal. In 2010, NPSG.02.02.01 was integrated into the Information Management standards as elements of performance 2 and 3 under IM.02.02.01.

Currently, this requirement does not apply to preprogrammed health information technology systems (for example, electronic medical records or CPOE systems), but this application remains under consideration for the future. Organizations contemplating introduction or upgrade of such systems should strive to eliminate the use of dangerous abbreviations, acronyms, symbols, and dose designations from the software.

Official "Do Not Use" List[1]

Do Not Use	Potential Problem	Use Instead
U, u (unit)	Mistaken for "0" (zero), the number "4" (four) or "cc"	Write "unit"
IU (International Unit)	Mistaken for IV (intravenous) or the number 10 (ten)	Write "International Unit"
Q.D., QD, q.d., qd (daily)	Mistaken for each other	Write "daily"
Q.O.D., QOD, q.o.d, qod (every other day)	Period after the Q mistaken for "I" and the "O" mistaken for "I"	Write "every other day"
Trailing zero (X.0 mg)*	Decimal point is missed	Write X mg
Lack of leading zero (.X mg)		Write 0.X mg
MS	Can mean morphine sulfate or magnesium sulfate	Write "morphine sulfate" Write "magnesium sulfate"
MSO_4 and $MgSO_4$	Confused for one another	

[1]Applies to all orders and all medication-related documentation that is handwritten (including free-text computer entry) or on pre-printed forms.

*Exception: A "trailing zero" may be used only where required to demonstrate the level of precision of the value being reported, such as for laboratory results, imaging studies that report size of lesions, or catheter/tube sizes. It may not be used in medication orders or other medication-related documentation.

The National Summit on Medical Abbreviations

Participants at the November 2004 National Summit on Medical Abbreviations supported the "do not use" list. Summit conclusions were posted on the Joint Commission website for public comment. During the four-week comment period, the Joint Commission received 5,227 responses, including 15,485 comments. More than 80 percent of the respondents supported the creation and adoption of a "do not use" list. This special one-day Summit brought together representatives of more than 70 professional societies and associations and special interest groups to discuss medical errors related to the misuse and misinterpretation of abbreviations, acronyms, and symbols. The objective of the Summit was to reach consensus on the scope and implications of this serious and complex problem and to find reasonable solutions using all of the evidence at hand and in the most dispassionate way possible.

The National Summit on Medical Abbreviations was hosted by The Joint Commission with its co-conveners American College of Physicians, American College of Surgeons, American Dental Association, American Hospital Association, American Medical Association, American Society of Health-System Pharmacists, Institute for Safe Medication Practices, and United States Pharmacopeia. Approximately 50 professional societies and associations and selected interest groups participated in the Summit representing every perspective.

For more information

Contact the Standards Interpretation Group at (630) 792-5900, or complete the Standards Online Question Submission Form at http://www.jointcommission.org/Standards/OnlineQuestionForm/.

APPENDIX E: POSTAL SERVICE ADDRESSING STANDARDS
TWO-LETTER STATE AND POSSESSION ABBREVIATIONS

Use the abbreviations below when transcribing or editing addresses. Using the two-letter state abbreviations makes it possible to enter the city, state, and five-digit ZIP Code (or ZIP+4 Code) on the last line of the address within 28 positions when necessary: 13 positions for city, one space between the city and state abbreviation, two positions for the state, two spaces (preferred) between the state and ZIP Code, and 10 positions for the ZIP+4 Code.

For further information on *Publication 28, Postal Addressing Standards*, go to the website at pe.usps.gov/cpim/ftp/pubs/Pub**28**/pub**28**.pdf.

State/Possession	Abbreviation
Alabama	AL
Alaska	AK
American Samoa	AS
Arizona	AZ
Arkansas	AR
California	CA
Colorado	CO
Connecticut	CT
Delaware	DE
District of Columbia	DC
Federated States of Micronesia	FM
Florida	FL
Georgia	GA
Guam	GU
Hawaii	HI
Idaho	ID
Illinois	IL
Indiana	IN
Iowa	IA
Kansas	KS
Kentucky	KY
Louisiana	LA
Maine	ME
Marshall Islands	MH
Maryland	MD
Massachusetts	MA
Michigan	MI
Minnesota	MN
Mississippi	MS
Missouri	MO
Montana	MT

State/Possession	Abbreviation
Nebraska	NE
Nevada	NV
New Hampshire	NH
New Jersey	NJ
New Mexico	NM
New York	NY
North Carolina	NC
North Dakota	ND
Northern Mariana Islands	MP
Ohio	OH
Oklahoma	OK
Oregon	OR
Palau	PW
Pennsylvania	PA
Puerto Rico	PR
Rhode Island	RI
South Carolina	SC
South Dakota	SD
Tennessee	TN
Texas	TX
Utah	UT
Vermont	VT
Virgin Islands	VI
Virginia	VA
Washington	WA
West Virginia	WV
Wisconsin	WI
Wyoming	WY

Geographic Directional	Abbreviation
North	N
East	E
South	S
West	W
Northeast	NE
Southeast	SE
Northwest	NW
Southwest	SW

Military "State"	Abbreviation
Armed Forces Europe, the Middle East, and Canada	AE
Armed Forces Pacific	AP
Armed Forces the Americas (except Canada)	AA

Military Address Formats

<u>Overseas military addresses</u> must contain the APO or FPO designation along with a two-character "state" abbreviation of AE, AP, or AA and the ZIP Code or ZIP+4 Code. The following examples show how the normal "city, state, zip" line would look when sending to a military base.

APO AE 09001-5275
FPO AP 96606-2783
APO AP 96522-1215

<u>Domestic Locations</u>

Use only the approved city name as listed in the City State file, along with the two-character state abbreviation and the ZIP Code or ZIP+4 Code as per example below.

MINOT AFB ND 58705-1253

APPENDIX F: UNITED STATES MILITARY BASES

United States Marine Corps (18)

Arizona	MCAS Yuma	Hawaii	MCB Hawaii
California	MCAGCC 29 Palms	North Carolina	MCAS Cherry Point
	MCLB Barstow		MCAS New River
	MCB Camp Pendleton		MCB Camp Lejeune
	MCAS Miramar	South Carolina	MCAS Beaufort
	MCRD San Diego		MCRD Parris Island
	Mountain Warfare Training Center	Virginia	Henderson Hall
Florida	MCSF Blount Island		MCB Quantico
Georgia	MCLB Albany	Washington, D.C.	Marine Barracks, Washington, D.C.

United States Navy (60)

California	NAWS China Lake	Nevada	NAS Fallon
	NB Coronado	New Jersey	NWS Earle
	NAS Lemoore		NAES Lakehurst, part of Joint Base McGuire-Dix-Lakehurst
	NPS Monterey	New York	NSA Saratoga Springs
	NAS North Island	Pennsylvania	NAS Willow Grove
	NB Point Loma	Rhode Island	NS Newport
	NB Ventura County-NAS Point Mugu	South Carolina	NSA Charleston
	NB Ventura County-NCBC Port Hueneme	Tennessee	NSA Mid-South
	Naval Base San Diego	Texas	NAS Corpus Christi
Connecticut	NSB New London		NAS JRB Fort Worth
Washington, D.C.	Washington NY		NS Ingleside
	United States Naval Research Laboratory		NAS Kingsville
Florida	Corry Station NTTC	Virginia	Chesapeake NSGA
	NAS Jacksonville		NSASP
	NAS Key West		Training Support Center Hampton Roads
	NS Mayport		NAB Little Creek
	NSA Orlando		NS Norfolk
	NSA Panama City		NAS Oceana
	NAS Pensacola		Wallops Island ASCS
	NAS Whiting Field		NWS Yorktown
Georgia	General Lucius D. Clay National Guard Center	Hawaii	NS Barking Sands
	NSB Kings Bay		Joint Base Pearl Harbor Hickam
	Dobbins ARB	Illinois	NS Great Lakes
Mississippi	NCBC Gulfport	Indiana	NSWC Crane Division
	NAS Meridian	Louisiana	NASJRB New Orleans
	NS Pascagoula	Maine	Portsmouth NS

Maryland	Fort Meade NSGA		NAS Whidbey Island
	NAS Patuxent River		NS Everett
	United States Naval Academy	West Virginia	NIOC Sugar Grove
Washington	NBK Bangor		
	NBK Bremerton		

United States Air Force (71)

Alabama	Maxwell Air Force Base	Nebraska	Offutt Air Force Base
Alaska	Clear Air Force Station	Nevada	Nellis Air Force Base
	Eielson Air Force Base	New Jersey	McGuire Air Force Base, part of Joint Base McGuire-Dix-Lakehurst
	Joint Base Elmendorf Richardson	New Mexico	Cannon Air Force Base
Arizona	Davis–Monthan Air Force Base		Holloman Air Force Base
	Luke Air Force Base		Kirtland Air Force Base
Arkansas	Little Rock Air Force Base	North Carolina	Pope Air Force Base
California	Beale Air Force Base		Seymour Johnson Air Force Base
	Edwards Air Force Base	North Dakota	Grand Forks Air Force Base
	Los Angeles Air Force Base		Minot Air Force Base
	March Joint Air Reserve Base	Ohio	Wright-Patterson Air Force Base
	McClellan Air Force Base	Oklahoma	Altus Air Force Base
	Travis Air Force Base		Tinker Air Force Base
	Vandenberg Air Force Base		Vance Air Force Base
Colorado	Buckley Air Force Base	South Carolina	Charleston Air Force Base
	Peterson Air Force Base		Shaw Air Force Base
	Schriever Air Force Base	South Dakota	Ellsworth Air Force Base
	United States Air Force Academy	Tennessee	Arnold Air Force Base
Delaware	Dover Air Force Base	Texas	Brooks City-Base
Washington, D.C.	Bolling Air Force Base		Dyess Air Force Base
Florida	Eglin Air Force Base		Goodfellow Air Force Base
	Hurlburt Field		Lackland Air Force Base, part of Joint Base San Antonio
	MacDill Air Force Base		Laughlin Air Force Base
	Patrick Air Force Base		Randolph Air Force Base, part of Joint Base San Antonio
	Tyndall Air Force Base		Sheppard Air Force Base
Georgia	Moody Air Force Base	Illinois	Scott Air Force Base
	Robins Air Force Base	Indiana	Grissom Joint Air Reserve Base
Hawaii	Joint Base Pearl Harbor Hickam	Kansas	McConnell Air Force Base
Idaho	Mountain Home Air Force Base	Louisiana	Barksdale Air Force Base
Mississippi	Columbus Air Force Base		New Orleans Joint Reserve Base
	Keesler Air Force Base	Maryland	Joint Base Andrews Naval Air Facility
Missouri	Whiteman Air Force Base	Massachusetts	Hanscom Air Force Base
Montana	Malmstrom Air Force Base		Westover Joint Air Reserve Base

Utah	Hill Air Force Base	Wyoming	Francis E. Warren Air Force Base
Virginia	Langley Air Force Base		
Washington	Fairchild Air Force Base		
	JBLM McChord Field, Joint Base Lewis-McChord		

United States Army Installations

This is a list of links for **U.S. Army** forts and installations, organized by U.S. state or territory within the United States. For consistency, major Army National Guard training facilities are included but armory locations are not.

- Alabama
  - Anniston Army Depot
  - Fort Rucker
  - Redstone Arsenal
- Alaska
  - Fort Greely
  - Fort Wainwright
  - Joint Base Elmendorf-Richardson
- Arizona
  - Camp Navajo (ARNG)
  - Fort Huachuca
  - Yuma Proving Ground
- Arkansas
  - Camp Joseph T. Robinson (ARNG)
  - Fort Chaffee Maneuver Training Center (ARNG)
  - Pine Bluff Arsenal
- California
  - Camp Beale
  - Camp Cooke
  - Camp Haan
  - Camp Roberts (ARNG)
  - Camp San Luis Obispo
  - Fort Hunter Liggett
  - Fort Irwin
  - Los Alamitos Joint Forces Training Base
  - Military Ocean Terminal Concord
  - Naval Base Point Loma
  - Parks Reserve Forces Training Area
  - Presidio of Monterey
  - San Joaquin Depot
    - Sharpe Facility
    - Stockton's Rough & Ready Island
    - Tracy Facility
  - Sierra Army Depot
- Colorado
  - Fort Carson
  - Fort Logan National Cemetery
  - Pueblo Chemical Depot
- Connecticut
  - Camp Niantic (ARNG)
- Delaware
  - Bethany Beach Training Site (ARNG)[1]
- District of Columbia
  - Fort Lesley J. McNair
- Florida
  - Camp Blanding (ARNG)
- Georgia
  - Camp Frank D. Merrill
  - Fort Benning
  - Fort Gordon
  - Fort Stewart
  - Hunter Army Airfield
- Hawaii
  - Fort DeRussy (MWR Resort)
    - Hale Koa Hotel
  - Fort Shafter
  - Kunia Field Station
  - Pohakuloa Training Area
  - Schofield Barracks
  - Tripler Army Medical Center
  - Wheeler Army Airfield
- Idaho
  - MTA Gowen Field Boise (ARNG)
  - Orchard Range TS Boise (ARNG)
  - TS Edgemeade Mountain Home (ARNG)
- Illinois
  - Charles M. Price Support Center
  - Rock Island Arsenal

- Indiana
  - Camp Atterbury
  - Fort Benjamin Harrison
- Iowa
  - Camp Dodge
  - Fort Des Moines
  - Iowa Army Ammunition Plant
- Kansas
  - Fort Leavenworth
    - Munson Army Health Center
  - Fort Riley
  - Great Plains Joint Training Area (ARNG)
    - Kansas Regional Training Institute (ARNG)
    - Nickel Hall Barricks (ARNG)
    - Smokey Hill Weapons Range (ANG)
- Kentucky
  - Blue Grass Army Depot
  - Fort Campbell
  - Fort Knox
- Louisiana
  - Camp Beauregard
  - Fort Polk
    - Peason Ridge Artillery Range
- Maine
  - MTA Deepwoods (ARNG)
  - MTA Riley-Bog Brook (ARNG)
  - TS Caswell (ARNG)
  - TS Hollis Plains (ARNG)
- Maryland
  - Aberdeen Proving Ground
  - Camp Fretterd Military Reservation (ARNG)
  - Fort Detrick
  - Fort George G. Meade
- Massachusetts
  - Camp Curtis Guild (ARNG)
  - Camp Edwards (ARNG)
  - Fort Devens
  - Natick Army Soldiers Systems Center
- Michigan
  - Camp Grayling(ARNG)
  - Detroit Arsenal
  - Fort Custer (ARNG)
- Minnesota
  - Camp Ripley (ARNG)

- Mississippi
  - Camp McCain (ARNG)
  - Camp Shelby
  - Mississippi Ordnance Plant
- Missouri
  - Camp Clark (ARNG)
  - Fort Leonard Wood
- Montana
  - Fort William Henry Harrison (ARNG)
- Nebraska
  - Camp Ashland (ARNG)
- Nevada
  - Hawthorne Army Ammunition Depot
- New Jersey
  - Fort Dix, part of Joint Base McGuire-Dix-Lakehurst
  - Picatinny Arsenal
- New Mexico
  - Los Alamos Demolition Range
  - White Sands Missile Range
- New York
  - Camp Smith (New York) (ARNG)
  - Fort Drum
  - Fort Hamilton
  - United States Military Academy at West Point
  - Watervliet Arsenal
- North Carolina
  - Camp Butner (ARNG)
  - Camp Davis
  - Camp Mackall
  - Fort Bragg
  - Military Ocean Terminal Sunny Point
- North Dakota
  - Camp Grafton (ARNG)
- Ohio
  - Camp Perry (ARNG)
  - Camp Ravenna Joint Military Training Center (ARNG)
  - Camp Sherman (ARNG)
- Oklahoma
  - Camp Gruber (ARNG)
  - Fort Sill
  - McAlester Army Ammunition Plant
- Oregon
  - Camp Rilea (ARNG)
  - Umatilla Chemical Depot

- Pennsylvania
  - Carlisle Barracks
  - Fort Indiantown Gap (ARNG)
  - Harrisburg Military Post (ARNG)
  - Letterkenny Army Depot
  - New Cumberland Army Depot
  - Tobyhanna Army Depot
- Puerto Rico
  - Fort Buchanan
  - San Juan Army National Guard Support Station
  - Camp Santiago
  - Fort Allen
  - Roosevelt Roads Army Reserve Base
- Rhode Island
  - Camp Varnum (Narragansett, RI) (ARNG)
  - Camp Fogarty (East Greenwich, RI) (ARNG)
- South Carolina
  - Fort Jackson
- South Dakota
  - Fort Meade (ARNG)
  - Tennessee
  - Holston Army Ammunition Plant
  - Kingston Demolition Range
  - Milan Army Ammunition Plant
- Texas
  - Camp Bowie
  - Camp Bullis
  - Camp Mabry
  - Camp Stanley Storage Activity
  - Camp Swift
  - Camp Wolters (ARNG)
  - Corpus Christi Army Depot
  - Fort Bliss
  - Fort Hood
  - Fort Sam Houston, part of Joint Base San Antonio
    - Brooke Army Medical Center

- Martindale Army Airfield
  - Red River Army Depot
- Utah
  - Camp W. G. Williams (ARNG)
  - Dugway Proving Ground
  - Tooele Army Depot
- Vermont
  - Camp Ethan Allen Training Site (ARNG)
- Virginia
  - Camp Pendleton State Military Reservation (ARNG)
  - Fort A.P. Hill
  - Fort Belvoir
  - Fort Eustis
  - Fort Lee
  - Fort McNair, part of Joint Base Myer-Henderson Hall
  - Fort Myer, part of Joint Base Myer-Henderson Hall
  - Fort Pickett (ARNG)
  - The Judge Advocate General's Legal Center and School
  - Quantico Military Reservation
  - National Ground Intelligence Center
  - Radford Army Ammunition Plant
  - Warrenton Training Center
- Washington
  - Joint Base Lewis-McChord
  - Yakima Training Center
- West Virginia
  - Camp Dawson West Virginia Training Area (ARNG)
- Wisconsin
  - Fort McCoy
  - Camp Williams (ARNG)
- Wyoming
  - Guernsey Maneuver Area (ARNG)
- U.S. states with no U.S. Army posts
  - New Hampshire
  - Rhode Island

APPENDIX G: RESOURCES

Accents
Interpreting ESL Medical Dictation. Modesto, CA: Health Professions Institute, 2008. http://www.hpisum.com and http://www.hpisum.com/ESLcdsContents.pdf

Office of Intramural Training & Education: https://www.training.nih.gov/us_english_resources

Purdue OWL Online Writing Lab: https://owl.english.purdue.edu/owl/

The Dialect Resource: http://dialectresource.com/

Voice and Speech Trainers Association (VASTA): http://www.vasta.org

Career Resources
AHDI Education Approval: <http://www.ahdionline.org/Careers/NewMTTraining/AboutEducation ProgramApproval/tabid/210/Default.aspx>

AHDI Model Curriculum for Healthcare Documentation: http://www.ahdionline.org/Careers /NewMTTraining/AboutEducationProgramApproval/tabid/210/Default.aspx#ModelCurriculum

Getting Your Foot in the Door: Two Years' Experience Not Required. Association for Healthcare Documentation Integrity: http://www.ahdionline.org

HelpGuide.org (information on interviewing): http://www.helpguide.org/life/interviewing_ techniques_tips_getting_job.htm

U.S. Department of Labor Statistics: http://www.bls.gov/ooh/healthcare/medical-transcriptionists .htm#tab-1

Just For Fun
Nichols, Kathy. *Bloopers, Typos, and Speech Wreck.* 2009.

CareerStep Medical Transcription blog: http://www.careerstep.com/blog/medical-transcription-news/speech-wreck-the-butt-of-the-joke and http://www.careerstep.com/blog/medical-transcription-news/speech-wreck-context-counts

Dr. Grumpy in the House (blog): http://drgrumpyinthehouse.blogspot.com/

Voice Tie Bows (blog): http://www.writeworks.biz/blog/voxrec/

Medical and Speech Recognition Errors and Case Studies
Agency for Healthcare Research and Quality: http://www.ahrq.gov/

U.S. Department of Health & Human Services: http://www.hhs.gov

Web M&M (Morbidity and Mortality): http://www.webmm.ahrq.gov/

Medical terms/drugs/abbreviations:
American College of Radiology, Glossary of MRI Terms: http://www.acr.org

Benchmark KB: https://benchmarkkb.interfix.biz

Drugs.com: http://www.drugs.com

MEDical ABBREViations: http://www.medabbrev.com

Lance, Leonard L. *Quick Look Drug Book.* Baltimore, MD: Lippincott, Williams & Wilkins, 2013. (In the alphabetical listing of drugs, pages 16–970, pronunciations are written in at each generic drug listing.)

RxList: http://www.rxlist.com

Drake, Ellen and Randy. *Saunders Pharmaceutical Word Book.* Philadelphia, PA: Elsevier, 2012.

U.S. Food and Drug Administration (FDA): http://www.fda.gov

Medical Videos (Diseases and Surgical Procedures)
Blausen Medical Communications, Inc: http://blausen.com/

OR Live: http://www.orlive.com/

Professional Associations:

American Health Information Management Association (AHIMA): http://www.ahima.org

Association for Healthcare Documentation Integrity (AHDI): http://www.ahdionline.org

Health Information Management Systems Society (HIMSS): http://www.himss.org

Health Story Project: http://www.himss.org/health-story-project

Physician Lookup:

http://www.ucomparehealthcare.com/drs/ – Find a doctor by state, specialty, or name. This website is also great for locating job openings.

http://www.healthgrades.com/ – Find doctors, dentists, and hospitals.

http://www.drscore.com/ – A website for measuring patient satisfaction. Patients can look up physicians and rate them with a score. Physicians can view summaries of their ratings using this site.

N.B.: Most physician names can be verified by searching online for the name of the hospital or clinic where they work, locating the "Find a Physician" area, and then searching by name or specialty.

Spellchecker Programs:

MediSpell Medical Spell Checker with Free Online Medical Speller

Spellex Medical and Pharmaceutical Spell Checker for Microsoft Word

Steadman's Plus 2014 Medical/Pharmaceutical Spell Checker

Technology:

A variety of proprietary transcription platforms are being used today. On-the-job training will be provided depending on the platform being used to transcribe medical records and the organization involved. While it certainly is not necessary to learn how to use every platform on the market, browsing the capabilities and functionality of various models will be helpful to keep up on current trends. Listed below are a handful of such platforms.

3M™ ChartScript™ Software: http://solutions.3m.com/wps/portal/3M/en_US/Health-Information-Systems/HIS/Products-and-Services/Products-List-A-Z/ChartScript-Software/

Nuance Dragon Medical 360/eScription: http://www.nuance.com/for-healthcare/dragon-medical-360/index.htm

EmDat InScribe: https://www.emdat.com/software/inscribe.asp

IntraScript: http://www.intrascript.com/

WebChartMD: http://www.webchartmd.com/

Word (Text) Expansion Programs:

Instant Text: http://www.fitaly.com/

Phrase Express Autotext for Windows: http://www.phraseexpress.com/

Smartype: http://www.smartype.com

SpeedType: http://www.speedtype.com/

Disclaimer: *Third-party products and services mentioned in this text are to enhance user's knowledge and awareness only. This is by no means an all-inclusive or complete list of products and services used in the healthcare documentation marketplace; the authors and publisher of this text endorse no particular product or service mentioned.*

APPENDIX H: BIBLIOGRAPHY

The American College of Radiology (ACR) website: http://www.acr.org

Association for Healthcare Documentation Integrity (AHDI). Accessed April 19, 2014. http://www.ahdionline.org/

The Book of Style for Medical Transcription, 3rd ed. Modesto, CA: Association for Healthcare Documentation Integrity, 2008.

Davis, N.M. *Medical Abbreviations: 32,000 Conveniences at the Expense of Communication and Safety,* 15th ed. Westminster, PA: Neil M. Davis Associates, 2010.

Diehl, M.O. *Medical Transcription Techniques and Procedures,* 7th ed. Philadelphia, PA: W.B. Saunders Company, 2012.

Dorland's Illustrated Medical Dictionary, 32nd ed., plus Dorland's online version. Philadelphia, PA: Elsevier, 2013.

Drake, E. *Sloane's Medical Word Book,* 5th ed. Philadelphia, PA: W. B. Saunders Company, 2011.

Drake, E. & Drake, R. *Saunders Pharmaceutical Word Book.* Philadelphia, PA: W. B. Saunders Company, 2012.

Lance, L.L. *Quick Look Drug Book.* Hagerstown, MD: Lippincott Williams & Wilkins, 2013.

The Merck Manual, 18th ed. Merck Research Laboratories, Whitehouse Station, NJ, 2006.

Merriam-Webster Online Dictionary. Accessed March 30, 2014. http://www.merriam-webster.com/dictionary/credentials

Merriam-Webster's Collegiate Dictionary, 11th ed. Merriam-Webster, Inc., Springfield, MA, 2006.

Phoenix, Jordan. *Uncommon Sense for 21st Century Living.* Accessed March 3, 2014. http://uncommonsense.is/

"Phonetics" definition. *Webster's New World College Dictionary,* 4th ed. Cleveland, OH: Wiley Publishing, Inc., 2002.

Postal Addressing Standards, Publication 28: United States Postal Service, November 2000.

Radiology Imaging, 2nd ed. Health Professions Institute, Modesto, CA, 2005.

Rice, J. *Medical Terminology: A Word Building Approach,* 7th ed. Upper Saddle River, NJ: Prentice Hall, 2010.

Stedman's Medical Dictionary, 28th ed. Baltimore, MD: Lippincott, Williams & Wilkins, 2006.

Stedman's Medical Dictionary for the Health Professions and Nursing, 5th ed. Baltimore, MD: Lippincott, Williams & Wilkins, 2005.

Stedman's Orthopedic & Rehab Words, 6th ed. Baltimore, MD: Lippincott, Williams & Wilkins, 2009.

Tessier, Claudia. *The Surgical Word Book,* 3rd ed. St. Louis, MO: Elsevier Saunders, 2004.

Truss, Lynn. *Eats, Shoots and Leaves.* New York, NY: Penguin Group (USA) Inc., 2004.

Turley, S.M. *Medical Language,* 2nd ed. Upper Saddle River, NJ: Prentice Hall, 2011.

The Wall Street Journal. *Pilots Rely Too Much on Automation, Panel Says.* Accessed April 19, 2014. http://online.wsj.com/news/articles/SB10001424052702304439804579204202526288042

Clark, Richard. *The Journal of the European Medical Writers Association.* "The Write Stuff," Vol. 2, No. 16, 2007.

General online resources consulted:

http://www.cancer.gov
http://www.cdc.gov/
http://www.drugs.com
http://www.mayoclinic.com
http://www.medabbrev.com
http://www.mtdesk.com
http://www.medicaltranscription.com/
http://www.ninds.nih.gov/
http://www.nlm.nih.gov/
http://www.rxlist.com
http://www.surgery.com/
http://www.webmd.com/
http://en.wikipedia.org/

INDEX